How toxic are my trousers?

AND

A guide on refining the senses to navigate the world of materials

The Uncut Edition

By Shaun M Sutton

How toxic are my trousers?
And a guide on refining the senses to navigate the world
of materials

The Uncut Version.

First Edition

ISBN 978-0-9576346-0-2

Written by Shaun M Sutton
Published by Herb Publishing
www.herbpublishing.com
Copyright © Shaun M Sutton 2013

Printed and distributed by Lightning Source
Book cover and design by Melanie Blumenthal at Herb Publishing.

I. Environmentally friendly architecture and product design.
II. Complimentary medicine. III. Popular psychology

Dedicated to

Ko Hung (283–343 AD) & Jack Kerouac (1922-69)
who may have been the same person in different lifetimes

Sharing a love for that same part of man,
sharing issue with the rest.
Men of old with shared observation,
who's to say those are times past
and not the same as now.

How Toxic are my trousers?

Parts I to X

A guide on refining the senses to navigate the world of materials
-to go sense and response friendly-

Appendices 1-8

All that matters

Standing out in the rain,
separate from the grass beneath my feet and the air I breath,
the babble of the hoards roam the shores of my mind,
harass the land within.

As the rain brings life to the earth,
and pencil joins the drops as I muse,
a cavern that exists is filled.
The gorge that was is crossed,
I'm back where I began.

To the world I'm fool in a red hat, standing in the rain,
that's fair play to say.
The air holds a pungency of smoke,
I guess from burning leaf pile in a garden somewhere over.

There is another existence,
stretching from my feet,
crossed by all things I need recognise.
All that was just now has no meaning to me,
when I wonder on what scheme matters.

The breeze refreshes like a storm,
the hoards are washed back to where they came,
my land is free to wander.
Antagonism as a memory is no more.

Preface

I met a buddy the other day, she was eating her favourite national snack food and asked if I'd like a taste. I took hold of a bag of Biltong, from South Africa, stepped outside, quietly response tested it in my own space, without any entering my mouth, and decided it was not for me. She said it didn't quite taste the way it was back home. The ingredients label was in small print so I asked her to read out loud to me the list of what was contained, beyond the cured meat. Gosh, no wonder my test lead me to turn down my first Biltong offering, all that rubbish added in to potentially make it no longer fit for my consumption. I suggested the best thing she could do was to bin it, throw it away. She however said she'd bought a big pack of it, from a really cool shop specialising in many of the familiar products from back home, and was all reluctant to follow my suggestion, partly due to the waste, and also, I'm guessing, because it connected her to the land she was missing and had left behind when she moved over seas to end up in London. I'm not sure if she followed my advice.

Is that it, the problem we are facing? Have we invested so much into what we live with now, and become overly connected to or caught up with the way we live and where we are coming from, it makes it hard to change, to let go of stuff, ways, scrap it and to start over again, to make a fresh beginning?

This work is about where and how to actually start off with the fresh beginning.

Introduction

A tale of discovery, for oneself

'Trousers', as I refer to this book, is about an enquiry made into the material world as a consequence of refining and developing my senses of perception. Starting out with my trousers and then moving onto other articles of clothing contained in the wardrobe, this work tells the tale of these explorations into clothing and then beyond, to question and consider a different view of the world, through engaging it more by way of using the senses and responses.

In the front half of the book is 'how toxic are my trousers?', a tale of my discovering of how to use the senses and experiences I had as a consequence. I do think of this as an exploration, beginning at my trousers, that's where my expedition into a somewhat hidden and alternate world happened to commence. At the rear half of the book is 'A guide on refining the senses to navigate the world of materials', also referred to as the appendices, detailing how to develop and be able to observe and use the senses and responses for oneself. In many ways these appendices could be of more value than the tale of my 'Trousers', however the two parts of the book are hopefully supportive of each other if one is to actually begin practising a more sense and response friendly way of life.

My investigations continue. Unfortunately I still don't have so many of the answers I am looking for, with possibly even more unanswerable questions. I'm left at a stage where I'm not exactly sure where it all goes from here on. It's a bit like having gone on a round the world tour for many months, or years even, you observe a different way of living and being, eat novel foods, have your experiences and stories to tell. Then making a return home, all that time later and the world we departed away from continues just as we left it, and we could even consider ourselves as being alien in our own home area where we grew up. Then is it back to the life we left off at, the job, the habits and lifestyle, leaving that across the seas to become some faded fabled dream world, and now we are back to business again as usual, working beyond our levels of comfort, doing the same as everyone else around us? Or, is it possible to make a change after our journey, improve ourselves without being sucked back into where it was we were before originally departing? In this particular case it is about departing the regular way of doing life, to begin exploring that which is immediate to us by way of just using the senses and responses, and see the behind the scenes world, glimpse something of the subconscious world affecting our being.

Going with the mainstream is very inviting. I think there are a lot of mainstream adults being forced by their situations to live with some level of delusion about how what we are doing in life is the way of things, even to the point of convincing themselves their way is the best to become fulfilled with oneself with some measure of success. Then we maybe try to sell ours as the optimal way and most admirable approach to life. Gosh sounds like me, no less deluded than the next person peddling their version of what life is about.

The problem for me, personally being someone open to the suggestion of others, is it is difficult to spot and work out who is telling the truth within their delusion, and so the world becomes either very complicated, forcing us to retreat into tried and tested ways and societal norms, or we can go out and try to work it out for ourselves, as I have attempted doing, providing the basis for this tale. The risk in departing the well trodden path is in getting lost in the woods and losing sight of where we are and what we are doing. Perhaps this tale will do that to you, leave you lost, cut adrift, sinking, hopeless and poor, without the means to support yourself according the ways you once knew. This I do not know, trying anything new out has some risk. Just the other day someone suggested to me that we have to get lost before we can develop, but I am not completely sure about this.

"Where's the dream vision, your promise Shaun, why should I go to the trouble of reading this work you've written on sense and response, or take any notice of it, I'm human, I naturally sense and respond?", I can almost hear these thoughts from some readers. Possibly then this is not a book for you, and you will not respond well to it, as I cannot make any promises you cannot keep, so I've tried to minimise the promise. As an alternative pledge I aim to avoid being too esoterically 'New Age', that's all I can promise in this work on exploring the senses and responses, I'm trying to keep this as real, tangible, touchable, and objective as I can, within limit.

There was this best selling book 'Celestine Prophecy', which was about following the signs and messages. I burnt my first copy at page 100, simply because it was coming across as overly esoteric for me, for want of a better expression and putting it kindly for the author and those who liked it. Somehow I ended up being given three or four copies of it over the years, by different people who thought it just the sort of book for me to read, so I'm not sure what that said about me back then. Putting it simply I've since gone down the path where I have to touch and feel to experience and believe. I think of 'Trousers' as being the story of venturing further along this touchy feely path than is usual to go down and explore what I find out there.

On the upbeat note what this work here hopefully provides is the means and tools to refine one's own senses and responses, our compass in navigation to making certain that key choices are good solid choices of consequence, then trying bring the matters raised during the expedition into a wider context concerning our world in general, at least that is my wish anyway. I may get there in the end, or I may lose you before that point, you maybe don't even reach beyond page 100.

I have attempted to write this work whilst in as good a general inner place as I can find, a place of peace and health, mostly found from being outdoors, and as close to the natural world as my location allows. Much of the work's structure at least began being written in draft form on my local bench by the River Thames during this summer just passed. Another title could almost have been, 'tales from a bench by the Thames'.

So as the reader is under no illusion on of the type of person I am, I feel it important to point out that I am no angel. I smoke and drink and party, although somewhat less than I used to. I am aware that these things are the vices of the era I grew up in and are not beneficial to good health. However, for whatever reasons I have continued to maintain some degree of these habits.

I live in the outskirts of London, just a 20 minutes rail journey from the city centre. I say this because certain aspects of what is included in this work could be more akin to that of a hermit living up in the mountains or forests, away from civilisation, which I am not. To all intents and purposes I am just a regular guy living in London, trying to make his way in life. I am no role model, I've just worked out how to use the senses and responses that's all, having been inspired on this direction as consequence of my being a student and practitioner of Traditional East Asian Medicine. My researching further into the senses likely came as a result of being influenced by the work of a group of practitioners in traditional medicine from Japan, itself as a country being originally influenced by the traditional medicine of China. In fact much of my own acupuncture practice and study was specifically developed by a group of partially sighted and blind acupuncture practitioners in Japan, also being a country where acupuncture had traditionally been promoted as a profession for the blind. This hopefully provides some insight to the background from where this is perhaps coming. I will say though that I have never had the pleasure of going to Japan to study this or anything else, and I am not sure this makes much difference to my tale. Maybe it does, through my being forced to develop somewhat separately from the source of the initial inspiration in my profession, with my coming from England.

I live between two quite distinct inner worlds, the chaotic and the peaceful, but have to function on the whole in the chaotic. The extent of the differences in these two worlds may be due to the cocktail of my life, of living in London, who I am, my past, my profession as a practitioner of Traditional East Asian Medicine, added with the influence of habits from my era.

I cannot help considering the nature of the experiences I describe are to some greater or lesser extent a reflection of me being sick or actually ill on some level, although I'm not presently aware of the medical name for the condition I may or may not have. An individual uneducated in the use of the senses may suggest, and even be accurate in their analysis, that I suffer some sort of elaborate neurosis. Equally, if I could have maintained something more of a continuous perfect health over the years, much of my own experiences and observations may never have been possible to witness.

This tale could also prove to be of some assistance for the individual seeking to discover what perfect health is, as much as in gaining an appreciation of how the ways we live, our environment, the personal materials, foods and things we live with, as well as our health care system all play their combined roles in supporting or denuding the processes of finding our perfect health state, as well as in recognising when we have found it.

My first herbal medicine teacher Michael Tierra once said, during our last class with him, that we should now just get on with giving people herbs, not to be scared, we will not kill anyone. I remained a bit sceptical and uncertain and ended up continuing my studies into oriental medicine upon his recommendation. I could suggest the same thing with using our senses, don't be scared, don't be put off from applying them or using them to assist in your decision making. But to

Shaun M Sutton

begin, use them as a support to other more tested means in the decision taking processes, and avoid relying on them exclusively until you've repeatedly proven to yourself that your senses can be truly trusted, and you've fully digested the content in the second half of this book, within the appendices, unless that is you are already a master in this matter.

Using the senses can help refine decision making and taking but used exclusively, and especially by the rookie or novice, can get one into all sorts of trouble and even be dangerous to ones health, so caution and care go hand in hand with using the senses and responses. The tale in the first half of this book, 'Trousers', tells something of this matter and of my own experiences, mistakes, difficulties and errors in judgment, which may be helpful as a support for others choosing to make the transition over to utilising the senses and responses more regularly within daily life.

I am unsure if others will share the same experiences or views as I in using the senses. In this tale I have included all those things leading me to make my comment, with summary of my reflections in the chapter 'Dilemma to change'.

The question remaining is on whether there exists a bold new world to be found through learning to apply the senses and responses, a world currently lost to our mainstream society? I wonder how much longer it will remain fairly hidden from public view, maybe forever, maybe it is not meant to be found, or is actually what we need to find but somehow it cannot be accessed. How this all appears will surely be much dependant upon the current place of the individual reader concerning their own capacity to apply the senses in making daily choices. Alternatively, it could be quite easy to determine this work as a simple piece of fiction, a delusion or merely a plain hoax of sorts.

This is a story that might be best understood when followed from beginning to end, in presentation of a new world view unfolding when applying the senses and responses, so do not expect to immediately find the blossom and fruit of it. I have no idea of how this work will be received by those I hope it may interest, as it remains the raw and uncut version, unedited, which I hope will add more than remove from what is my intention to portray. Welcome to the world revealed by the senses and responses.

How toxic are my trousers?

Parts I to X

'The left leg'

Part I

My trousers, and the discovery of how toxic they were

"The radial pulses on the wrist are like a window, through which the core of a person can be viewed. They are a means of education, to teach ourselves about ourselves, about what goes on inside us, and how this compares with what's going on in the more visible aspects of our self"

In order to get to the point of gauging the toxicity of my trousers and the world extending beyond these, one needs a reference point to work from, call it 'my marker and gauge for toxicity about me'. The markers I use are not those utilising information provided by modern scientific research, although I imagine the markers I use could be of support in confirming scientific findings. I have a friend, Thomas in Germany, a structural engineer who upon learning of the title for this book, told me that in Germany there's a state department dedicated to the investigation of toxicity in materials, and that clothing is considered to be one of the key sources of toxicity in our personal environment. The department is the same one dealing with the annual testing of motorcars for road worthiness, the TÜFF, which is like the MOT in the UK.

As an acupuncturist and practitioner of Traditional East Asian Medicine I have found there are a variety of diagnostic techniques to guide practice. Of these diagnostic tools, in providing assistance to confirm how to treat each individual patient and monitor progression during the treatment process, is the measurement and consideration of the radial pulse quality at the wrist. Pulse taking remains of continual fascination to me personally and in the course of my professional work.

Many books have been written on the subject of pulse diagnosis, many of them very ancient. My problem, along with translating the pulse qualities into a diagnosis and treatment plan, partially because I may have been asleep in that particular lecture and always a possibility if it fell after lunch or on a Monday, was that I could not remember even a few of the rules described about the different pulses detailed in these books, or anything the pulse signified in terms of treatment, no matter how many times these were reviewed. A Chinese practitioner teacher of mine said that as a student in China he had to know the ancient pulse texts by

1

heart, and that he had learnt them sung as a song in his classes.

So pulse taking in my earlier days of practise essentially became limited to checking the pulses of my patients before treatment, and then periodically during the session to monitor how they changed during my work. I would like to add, in my defence as a practitioner who had been unable to read the pulses according to tradition, that pulse taking is just one of the means of diagnosis available to generate a treatment approach in oriental medicine, although it is a pretty main one.

I became somewhat of a pulse taking geek, not just in checking the pulse changes and qualities during the acupuncture and massage treatments I provided, but also feeling my own pulses and finding what influenced them when treating myself. As I could not remember the pulse texts by heart, I resorted to following my own simplified system to consider the overall pulse character, as well as the nature of changes in the pulse qualities, in comparison to the other changes being observed in my patients, or in me when trying out the therapies on myself.

During early experiments on myself, and on what would change my pulses, I realised how my thought pattern could change the character of the pulses whilst simply staring out of the window. If I focused on the trees in the garden for instance, and the green of their leaves, the shades and patterns, in a state of blissful wonderment of some form and then re-checked my pulses, they had become more gentle and quiet to me. Then whilst still staring out of the window I engrossed myself with thoughts of all the things I had to do, work related things, such as completing my tax return and day to day management matters for my business or personal commitments. The change in thought made the radial pulses become a bit faster with an element of hardness, even a pointedness in them, quite different in character to the easy relaxed rolling along of my earlier green moment pulses. (For further information on observing the pulse see appendix 1)

For some time in the treatment room, I had been playing with my own form of kinesiology in testing herbs against a patient's pulses, having been aware of the muscle tests performed by chiropractors in the USA, with a few similar aims, to determine a prediction of a patient's favourable to a remedy through simply them holding or touching it. I thought maybe I would be able to make similar predictive observation through, instead of muscle testing, just taking the pulses of patients whilst they were being introduced to remedies, as a supporting approach to the regular theories in selecting and prescribing herbs. Sometimes I thought I noticed something, but then on retesting often felt there was not really a notice-able positive response. My own state of mind and mental ease seemed to inter-fere with these test responses, and even though I was testing the pulses of my patients, how I was myself played its own part in affecting the pulse responses I was observing.

However, I continued playing with the notion that I could predict the nature of any response to a herb though the pulses. This was simply done by placing the herb container, with the herbs inside, in the patient's hand or on their tummy or back, on top of the covering sheet. Some patients were able to give me their own feedback to say things such as that one made the chest tight or they felt a bit sick, or this one felt ok by comparison. But overall it was a bit haphazard just relying on the pulse changes and I felt I could not completely rely on this as the fool proof system of working I was seeking, however I did continue observing and investigating the pulse to this end all the same.

I had spent some years learning Qi gong, a form of ancient Chinese calisthenetic, and practiced what I had learnt most days, finding a nice place outdoors on some grass, or in the woods, where ever I was that day. As a continuance of me being a pulse geek, I developed the habit of testing my pulses before and after my Qi gong exercises to observe their effect on my system according to the view I was considering them from.

In the summer of just over three years ago, my wife and myself travelled to Frankfurt in Germany to visit her friends and family. Frankfurt is quite a built up city, with not that many open green spaces directly within the city itself. We were staying with a friend in an older part of the city centre, just off the Schweizer Strasse. The morning sun and city noises woke me a little on the early side after a late night out in our favourite traditional Frankfurt restaurant. Sporting a some-what fuzzy head from too much Apfelwine, a local form of traditional cider, and one too many Mispelchen, a fruit preserved in Calvados apple brandy, I set out to find my green space in the sun for that morning's Qi gong, and to hopefully sort my head out, not quite sure of where to go.

Walking down the Schweizer Strasse, towards the River Maine, I came to the museums area, and found what I was looking for in the grounds of the Museum fur Kunsthandwerk (practical art museum). A couple of winos trawled the rub-bish bins for whatever it was they were looking for, so I chose my sunny position in the middle of the museum's grounds, far enough away from these undesirable looking characters for my safety and quietude. I do admit that I took off my shirt and sandals to exercise in only my combat style shorts, the type with deep pockets. Being shirtless in public places is perhaps a particularly English thing to do, and did nothing for hiding my presence to passers by, although walking via the tramps perhaps appeared more favourable than via a shirtless me performing my ancient Chinese calisthenetic.

At the end of my exercises I re-checked my pulses and it appeared that in spite of my best efforts at sorting myself out, the pulses remained quite hard and un-relaxed as compared to what I would generally observe from my own handy work at the end of the exercises at home. Maybe the affect of the previous evening's alcohol intake was still playing a part in this, stewed from the night before. After persisting a little longer to try to resolve the pulses through my exercise, whilst enjoying the brilliant morning sun on my skin, I thought about giving up and going back without any success, other than in getting a nice tan. It was at this point that I realised I was carrying the equivalent to the contents of a man bag within these long pockets of my shorts, so I took everything out and laid it all at my feet, whilst checking upon the location of the marauding wino tramps.

In my pockets included what one would generally carry when travelling. I preferred using my pockets for security reasons over a bag, partly because I am prone to putting things down and forgetting them. Passport, mobile phone, wallet, a big set of many keys, tobacco and lighter, my watch and loose change were all on the grass next to me. I then rechecked my pulses to find they were noticeably calmer, more relaxed and lacking the hardness apparent before the empty out. I then tried returning each set of these items individually into my pockets and retested the pulses to find that in each instance, except for the passport, my pulses had to some extent become harder once more, becoming relaxed once again on removing the articles.

Significant in these tests was my pulse response to the loose change and my keys, items I generally always carried on my person. This soon led to a full and thorough investigation on my part back home, of the metals on and about my person in regard to their affect on my pulses.

During this particular trip to Germany I had been celebrating my birthday. Some close friends of ours, we had travelled on to visit with in the south of Germany, presented me with a special birthday present, a lovely Lamy fountain pen, even engraved with my name on it. Back at home whilst writing my journal by the Thames in the evening with the new pen, I realised it made my pulses harder when I held it in my hand. It had a metal body.

The case of this pen is significant, for it became one of the very early casualties during my quest to rid myself of as much metal as possible. Sorry Ekey and Nicki, it was a thoughtful gift, and considerate of my enjoyment in writing stories, but it played its part in this story and so served a good use in making a point here, upon the extent I was attempting to remove as much metal as I feasibly could from being used in my immediate world.

In consideration of our day to day use of metals, testing of the contents of my trousers suggested that metal formed a potentially insidious and hard to exclude part of our daily life. And of course my trousers encompass the wholesale utilisation of metals in their make up, from the metal buckle of the belt to zippers, fastenings and bits holding materials together. Living without metal close to my person was going to be a difficult matter to overcome.

Back at home in London, I made a number of tests against my pulses of all the daily utilised metals, believing certain to make my pulses harder than others when in contact with my skin or close to my person. Beginning from as neutral place I could safely achieve, in my underpants, I made tests of all my trousers and decided that whilst I had to continue using metals, I would try to avoid those trousers whose metals I felt unsettled the equilibrium of my pulses more than others. I even took keys made of these certain metals to the key maker to have them cut in a more favourable metal for me, as far as I was able to perceive.

I then had the problem of those trousers being selected as acceptable, according to their metals content, were now few and the best of these were a little on the wide side for me. Now that I considered my belt to be a no-no, I had to walk about with the top of my trousers rolled over so they would not so easily slip off from my hips.

During this one particular weekend my wife had been busy away with friends, allowing me time to create as much mayhem as I needed in performing my trouser and metal tests in private. I don't think she would have allowed my weird frivolity if she had been around just at that time. Anyway, so I thought I could go out and find a much needed belt for myself, that better agreed with my pulses, with this momentary freedom from the watchful eye of my wife. I ventured out to make my very first shopping expedition, whilst using my pulses to guide my potential purchase, for a new pulse friendly belt in my local high street.

The High Streets in England tend to have all the same shops as each other, the High Street 'Names', perhaps this is an international phenomenon. All the main clothing stores were fairly close to each other, so I went to each and tried out testing their belts and buckles for the effect of their different metals on my pulses. Holding the buckle in one hand, I used the other to take my radial pulse, whilst trying to steady my mind in the midst of a busy Saturday for shoppers, or alternatively I was trying out the idea of putting the belt loosely around my waist to make this easier and have a free hand. It was quite difficult as I had to keep an eye out for the store employees who were asking me if I needed any help, whilst regularly pulling up my sagging jeans in order to not reveal and expose myself in public. I took trophy photographs of myself using our mobile phone camera in one store with a wonderfully wide selection of belts, holding up the one I felt was the best in front of the belt stand, like the proud hunter with his catch.

I visited one store twice that afternoon, but on this second visit, whilst trying to decide between a galvanised belt buckle with a superman logo on it over a more nonchalant and less obtrusive belt without motif, a store employee came up to me, whilst I was lingering and looking all shifty about the belt stand, and asked if I was sure I really didn't need any help, suggesting I'd been there for quite some while now. With alarms of panic in me about being found out for testing or worse, I decided to cut my losses and leave empty handed, the sun was out and I was feeling a bit exhausted by the whole belt testing shopping affair.

I would have to make do with my sagging jeans, which I then washed extra hot to try to shrink them enough to sit tighter upon my waist. When my wife returned home I proudly informed her of my adventures and mentioned about the concerns of the staff in the gents clothing department, which I had felt was funny. She was not amused in the slightest and told me off. "This town is too small for this sort of nonsense", her tone and words in reality a little stronger than this. When she later found the photos of me standing by the belt stand she was beginning to get a little more concerned about where this was going.

Part II

New world, pitfalls and uncertainty

To suddenly begin questioning the fabric of one's material world, in consideration of its neutral or negative influence upon how I was maybe feeling, lead me down a path of uncertainty on just about every thing one interacts with on a daily basis.

This is a matter of how open could the mind be to the extent of toxicity in my world, toxicity I was gauging by way of reading my pulses. At this point I was only just beginning to develop some basic awareness of the interaction of my body with the world. The pulses held their limitation as a tool of toxicity determination, especially in public places, as I had to hold my wrist for a while to read my pulses, which according to my wife, made me look really odd and dodgy. However, upon my discovery of a potential for pulse to environment correspondence phenomenon, I was drawn to investigating my environment further through making observation of the pulses.

My initial focus had been on metals, and whether certain metals on my person would cause a tightening and hardening of my pulses by comparison to others. Metals are used everywhere in our world. Certain of them definitely seemed less favourable according to my pulse measurement, although I am apprehensive to say which in case it's all just me, and because this is more a tale about the experience than theory I hope, and of learning how to use the senses as opposed to just believing anything some fool (like me) suggests. I believe that's the right idea?

So the long and short of it is that I did not use certain metals where ever I could avoid these and had option to use something I considered more favourable, or uncompromising of myself, as far as I was perceiving it. This lead me to stowing away a number of clothing articles, mostly trousers, for future potential tests in case I was to later feel the urge to test them again, rather than just dispose of them completely at this early stage.

A number of trips to my local second hand clothing stores replenished my wardrobe with articles I felt more comfortable about wearing, and provided me a particular new interest in clothing that I'd not experienced previously. This was much to the surprise of my wife, who knew me as someone not especially concerned about clothes. It was obvious to her I was beginning to change as a person, in good ways and bad, but I'm not sure which way was the most apparent that I might be going to her.

I began developing theories for my own guidance of what was acceptable to use against my skin, whilst I improved my wardrobe according the pulse responses.

The influence of these early theories began to percolate into the operation of both my personal and professional life. In the treatment room I removed all metal objects and electrical equipment from my immediate working space where this was an option. As an acupuncturist I even ceased using the metal acupuncture needles defining my profession, for concern over their affect on me, even with the rest of the world having no problems with the idea of using metals. My professional colleagues were somewhat entertained by my notion and questioning in this matter of 'could using needles be unhealthy for us working in the profession?'. (There exist many ways an acupuncturist can treat the body, and the modern acupuncture needle is in fact a fairly recent invention and more modern development).

My wife on the other hand was becoming concerned over my mental state and obsession with changing our flat about to suit my theories, theories that I was making up and could not prove to her. She was particularly perturbed by my refusal to use the expensive designer chairs due to their use of metal for the legs. I wanted as much natural material as I could conveniently and inexpensively utilise. I am ashamed to admit there were occasions where my obsession for the natural led to argument between us because I was ignoring her pleas to calm down and stop changing everything, which was of course affecting her too. In some ways it was harder for her as she did not understand my theories or particularly want to know anything of them. Once or twice she did scream in frustration something along the lines of "I cannot hear your toxic one more time, no more toxic!"

I cannot say how we managed it, it's a bit of a blur phase, but we made the changes I was requesting, our relationship did survive 'me and my toxic', and our home did improve. Gradually she came around to allowing me my idiosyncrasy for natural and non-toxic materials alternative to that of the synthetic world. All metals had to be restricted where ever possible, some more than others. That's where we were at in this all.

I began testing my theories out on friends, and some patients once I discovered the sorts of things they carried in their pockets or lived close by to in their homes, with varied and inconsistent results. That threw me and encouraged me. Newer theories replaced the old to help me make some sense of this new world I was waking to or just making up as I went along.

In testing, I found some people were not showing any response to the keys and money in their pockets, disproving any theory that all metal was bad for the pulse quality. One friend however, Thomas the structural engineer in Germany, slept with all the power tools of his trade under his own bed for lack of space in the apartment, which of course horrified me. So I treated him in his home and at the end of the treatment, when his pulses were nicely relaxed and softer, I brought in all the boxes of tools from his bedroom, about ten or so, and stacked them up around and under the treatment table where he was lying and quietly resting.

His pulses became noticeably harder and tighter from this, but when I then moved these tools away from the table, and re-stacked them to the side of the area where we were working in his lounge, his pulse returned to the previous more comfortable and relaxed character. After our test he commented that he too felt a difference in himself taking place during the test, whilst he lay there on his back with his eyes shut, only partially aware of what I was doing, although the clanking and rattling of the heavy cases to some extent gave this away.

He did move all his tools as a result of this test to a more distant location from his bed. He still does not wear a metal buckled belt for his trousers, which I was surprised to hear about when just recently he informed me of this. Also his chronic back problem cleared up completely, which may have been related. It is amazing how much trust we tend to place in the opinion other people and can believe almost anything we are informed about. Maybe in this instance he had good reason to believe me, but I am not he so I don't know.

Interestingly to me, his wife said she never liked the idea of sleeping with all the tool boxes under their bed. This kind of comment has been similarly made by my own wife at times when I've mentioned a new discovery leading to me no longer wearing an item of clothing I'd formerly lived out of. "I never liked you in that" she would say. Women perhaps have a deeper sense in these matters, although both his and my own wife trained as designers, which of course may make them more sympathetic naturally to how things should be. A female or designer's sixth sense in such matters, having the eye for how things look and feel, without needing to perform these elaborate tests of my own to bring us all to the same conclusion.

One time I did manage to demonstrate to my wife, and a friend Malcom at his house, of how my pulses responded to any coins in my pockets. First, without any items in my pockets I had each of them take a wrist and feel my radial pulse, pressing down and up to get a sense of how it felt to them. Then I had them place a quantity of British pound coins into my pocket and observe for themselves how my pulses became less relaxed, harder and more forceful. When they removed the coins from my pocket the pulses regained their former calmer and more relaxed quality. They both indicated they were able to observe these changes. It's not easy to demonstrate this sort of thing, let alone establish a greater relevance of meaning to it, beyond it appearing as merely an odd magic trick one could play.

The question remained for me that I somehow initiated the responses myself due to my anxieties over metals, in the same fashion I could change my pulses at will when looking out of the window into the garden during my earlier green pulse experiments. For instance could these anxieties even transfer from one to another person, like to my friend Thomas when I was testing him for power tools, giving the poor guy the impression that his trade's tools are toxic to him, when in fact it's just me affecting him as I'm standing right next to the pile of tools I'm testing him for?

During these early experimental days I have to admit that we were not sleeping on the healthiest of beds, an inflatable camping mattress for space saving purposes. However as chance would have it, this proved to be useful in making some further discoveries through good fortune coming out of poor circumstance.

One morning on waking, as I lay on the inflatable bed, I found my feet were hanging off the end of the mattress with my cotton socked feet resting on the wooden floor. I was looking out of our tall old fashioned sash windows, observing the plate sized leaves on the big London Plain trees growing outside the apartment. Through each window pain I could just see one limited section of the tree and it's lovely broad leafy foliage. I'm not certain of why I decided to perform my pulse tests with my heels on the floor and then again with my feet not touching the floor, but I did it and was surprised to discover that not only were my pulses harder and less relaxed when the heels were not touching the floor, but also I felt certain I could see more clearly the leaves through the window with my heels touching the floor. (During this test I need to say that I moved up in the bed to support my feet to be off the ground, rather than just lift them up, which would have activated the muscles and possibly change the pulses via the extra body tensions.)

Playing around I tried counting just those leaves I was able to clearly distinguish through one window pain and make comparison between the number I could count with heels touching the floor, and then again with my heels on the mattress. I reckoned I could more visibly see double the number of leaves with my heels touching the floor.

One of the bed socks I was wearing had a big hole in its heel. Somehow I then observed that only when the holed sock foot heel was touching the floor I was able to achieve this dramatic improvement in pulse and the quality of my vision. When only the other foot's heel touched the floor, which again by sheer chance had no hole in the sock's heel, the pulses hardened somewhat and it felt like the vision became less clear once again. As mentioned the bed socks were made of cotton.

These observations lead me to develop a variety of new tests and theories as a result, concerning the idea of an earthing of the body occurring through certain materials and not so much or at all through others. It appeared that certain materials insulated this earthing phenomenon from occurring, leading to these improvements in my vision, and my pulses to soften and relax.

Each morning for a while, whilst my wife hopefully remained asleep at my side on the inflatable mattress, I would conduct further 'earthing' experiments by placing a variety of materials by my side of the mattress on the wooden floor, laid out so I could easily place my fingers upon each test article, in a fashion allowing me to still observe changes in the radial pulses, and try to make out how many London Plain tree leaves I could clearly see through the window pain for each of the materials tested. This was quite some test to successfully perform.

According to my theories at that time, plastics prevented this earthing effect, observable through my pulses, which provided the reason the inflatable mattress facilitated observing these earthing benefits from my just touching the floor. Cotton to me became viewed a semi-insulator from my tests with jeans and T shirts at my bed side by improving the pulses to some degree, whereas putting my fingers on an item made of wool, such as my woollen jumper laid on the wood floor by the mattress, had pretty well the same affect on my pulses as me directly touching just the wooden floor at my mattress side. This really was a complete revelation to me. I tested, re-tested, blind tested to some degree, all whilst lying on my inflatable camping mattress in the mornings.

These bedroom experiments continued. Getting up as quietly as one can, from an inflatable mattress on a wooden floor, without disturbing the other person, my wife, it squeaking about on the wood when there was too much movement in getting off and on it, coming back to bed with handfuls of articles and materials to lay on the wooden floor to be tested for earthing qualities, as measurable by taking my pulses. Books with all sorts of different covers, leather, linoleum and various flooring tiles, ceramic tiles, pieces of slate, stones and rocks, snippets of material and fabrics I was collecting, shoes and boots, rope, shopping bags, china, crockery and glass of different form and manufacture. Each morning I would test five or so items of a particular test grouping. I made little notes of each of my pulse response observations to these, recording responses like a child might collect the sports personality cards coming free with a purchase of bubble gum. I just could not show my collection off to the world, far too geeky really even for me. My wife was trying to turn a sleeping blind eye to this, anxious over the prospect of what could be the next phase I would go through.

Whilst I have mentioned my wife did have her melt down moments over my toxic, I would try to stay calm and not react during the heat of the moment. I knew what I was doing was on the edge of familial acceptability, messing about as I was, testing this and that around the house. I just did my best to convince her that I was not harming her, or anyone else. I admit my behaviour could have been annoying to live with. That I did not retort to her occasional outward anger and anxieties towards me over my testing and changing things was surprising though, as I have been prone to angry retort in the past. But not now, this must not become an issue I felt, I just wanted to peacefully test my world and I had to be peaceful to test my world. I could not test my world without an empty and peaceful mind, this is the prerequisite I found necessary for the testing. I listened to my wife's feedback, took it on board, thinking maybe there was a point and that should mark the end of a particular testing phase. If she was becoming especially annoyed by me it was possible I was getting a little over obsessive with it all.

However the experiments continued, just as new ones. I cut holes in the heal of a few pairs of white cotton sports socks, as I had no woollen ones to hand, other socks I cut the elasticated top part from them, as I thought this was stopping my circulation somehow and was making the pulses harder for some reason. I then managed to locate and dig out a couple of pairs of old woollen hiking socks I had in storage, and then cleared out all the cotton socks from my drawer, including my recently doctored pairs, and chucked them all. It was nice to have an empty drawer also. I then continually lived out of just these two pairs of long black woollen socks.

What was amazing is that wool socks don't actually get so smelly as cotton, which is general knowledge I was not aware of, and do not need the daily change as with the cotton ones, which of course may not sound that inviting. But finding replacement new woollen socks without them being some sort of blend with synthetic material or costing the earth or looking ridiculous was not easy, so I just kept alternating the two pairs I had, hand washing them regularly until they completely lost their heals. They had really served me well and were like a couple of trusted old friends in the end.

One sunny day, after being inspired through observing some difference in myself whilst wearing rubber soled sandals in the garden after my Qi gong exercises, I performed my earthing tests outside in the back garden through carrying outdoors a plastic storage box lid to put my feet on. Whilst sitting on a plastic chair I was able to compare my pulses between being barefoot on the grass, or with my feet on the plastic lid, the chair and the lid both disconnecting me from the ground. The pulses were more relaxed and less forceful when the feet were direct to grass.

When out and about in a cafe or the cinema, or where there was a vinyl floor covering or on certain types of carpet, I'd sit and secretly touch the wall with my hand or bare elbow, or pushing a wooden chair against the wall or skirting board, so that I could touch or rest my leather boot upper against the chair, which via this contact route to the wall, enabled me to earth, through the wood to earth connection. My wife often knew what I was up to and could observe my weirdness in behaviour, but to the rest of the world hopefully there was nothing obvi-

Shaun M Sutton

ous going on with me whilst I tried to remain unobtrusive during my earthing activities in public places.

Leather, I deduced from my pulses, was a good material for earthing through. I had an old pair of Redwing brand boots that I lived out of which had a rather worn rubber sole to them that could be changed for leather at the shoe repairers. I was very excited by the possibility of being able to test whatever I walked on for it's earthing properties via new leather soles, I was desperate for that opportunity, fascinated I was with working out my world. I tried to explain to the shoe repairer that it had to be leather from sole to foot but could not explain to him the exact details of why, otherwise I fear I would have disconcerted the poor guy and have had an embarrassing moment. I was trying to behave all normal without giving my game away to ensure I could save face.

The long and short of it ended as the new leather soled pair being now better than they had been before with the rubber for earthing, but I noticed a rubber layer between the inner and outer sole which the repairer had stitched through. I think the stitching helped earth through the inner to the outer sole somewhat to allow something, but it was not a full earthing sole as it should have been as far as I was able to measure and gauge, meaning my pulses were still better if I were barefooted. In spite of this being a disappointment on my expectation, the new leather soled boots helped in identifying walking surfaces which did not allow my earthing phenomenon to occur through. I discreetly asked Graham the boot repairer, at the next re-sole, if it could be leather to leather as he had previously shown me a composite leather material which was to go between the inner and outer leather, but he said that the rubber part needed to remain for techie shoe repairer reasons.

I never imagined it would be so complicated a matter changing my rubber sole to an earthing leather one. In a way this is a reflection of the whole process of trying to make the changes in my world in order to help improve my pulses. I was speaking a different language and had different needs to everyone else. I felt like a new breed of vegan and the rest of the world were more like gourmet French chefs, from whom I wanted to ask if they could cook me a three course dinner but excluding the use of any animal or dairy product. I had to remain careful of explaining my reasons for being such a fussy and particular new breed to avoid any awkward questions I did not wish or maybe could not answer without panicking myself and confusing others.

One significant success however did arrive into my wife's and my life, a new futon to replace the inflatable mattress. I had contacted the Centre for Alternative Technology in Wales for any information they had on natural beds, as I could not get much success making Internet searches for more natural bedding. They recommended a company making their own futons and mattresses using all natural components. On contacting the company they were kind enough to send me samples of each of the materials used in the futon layers and a variety of cotton coverings (which were for my own earthing tests). I had wanted to use a linen cotton blend we had in a sample, but it was not durable enough for a cover. That particular blend had felt better on the pulses from off the inflatable mattress, more so than the pure or organic cotton material snippets during these early 'Earth to Shaun' experiments.

So this was progress, and at last my tests where having an effect on improving our lives, fruit from my labours and my wife's patience. However we could not afford the new natural organic bed quilts, quilt covers, or pillows and their cases to go with the futon. Progress could only go so fast. The most important thing was that change was happening, with the foundation for these changes coming from the point of view of my own senses. A step toward a potentially doubtful and dubious new world based purely on my own responses and what I had made of them. This was a new form of DIY.

At this time my wife and I were toying with the idea of moving to Frankfurt in Germany, her home city. The idea was for her to be closer to her professional connections in Design and the colleagues she had studied with at that City's University of Design in Offenbach. Some friends were kind enough to let us stay at their nice apartment in Bornheim, a trendy part of Frankfurt, for a few months whilst they travelled to Australia. We ended up living between London and Frankfurt for almost a year whilst investigating our home location options, suck each and see how we felt about where to base ourselves in the future.

During these visits to Bornheim the experience of sleeping in a real bed meant that I could not sleep with my foot off the futon and touching the floor, a habit I had developed with the inflatable mattress and maintained even with the new futon as I felt it still better for my pulses. So I pulled up an old wooden stool next to the bed, and rested my hand on it whilst I fell asleep to make a contact through it to the wooden floor. Yes, certainly obsessive, compulsive maybe. I mention this to show the extent of my concerns and the uncertainty developing about my world when I began questioning the affect of the fabric of the material world in which I lived. For me it often felt disconcerting, detaching myself from the regular ways of accepting things as generally accepted and to try out living according to what my own body was informing me of. This lead me often towards what I now consider as barmy acts, when I became unsure about almost everything, in the hope I could somehow cling on to sanity through earthing myself. Sleeping with my hand on a stool seemed quite an acceptable thing to consider at the time and really, it made me feel calmer and sleep more easily. You can think it, that's OK, barking crazy.

I felt inquisitive and interested to learn what I could for myself and quite surprisingly I did not feel like I was on the edge of breakdown, more on the edge of a breakthrough! This could be the sort of thing someone with Bipolar Syndrome may of course say during a manic episode, so it was more unsettling for my wife than for me. But somehow she let me get on with my silly stuff. I wasn't much of a public menace or at risk of harming myself and was not showing any outward indication of mania, just a bit of tiredness and a regular inability to easily sleep at night perhaps.

Our friends' apartment in Germany got a work over by us to make it a little more response friendly to live in. They had been sleeping with a big metal cabinet directly at the end of their bed, upon which sat a massive old fashioned TV set. This time both of us were shocked at our friends sleeping and living situation, which needed changing, so we isolated the sleeping area from all metals and electric devises. There was me thinking that I am the crazy one here, then I see how other people live and question who are the crazy ones? Yet the next tale may provide a different perspective on this matter of my crazy, and the barmy and obsessive acts.

Some close friends of ours were getting married and planned a wedding party in what was virtually a castle in the former East Germany, between Hamburg and Berlin. This was some sort of old ancestral house, I'm guessing built in the 17th or 18th Century, recently restored to much of its former level of glory and now converted into a Hotel. Perfect for anyone who wants to experience the grandeur of a stay in a castle and the fairy tale weddings venue.

Our room was beautifully put together, and quite expensive for us on our budget, not even able afford new pillows on our own bed at home. Never mind. But it was a special occasion, and the duty was on us to attend. Whilst my wife was in the bathroom, showering and getting ready for our first evening's celebration, after our all day long and hot drive across the length of Germany, I decided to re-address the sleeping area, the bed and various aspects of the room, according to my pulses and senses.

When she came out cleaned up and getting dressed up for our evening event she almost screamed at me, horrified at what I had made of this previously perfectly presented antique hotel bedroom. I'd pulled the mattresses off the bed and stacked them at the end of the room. I had tested the bed and felt it better to sleep on just the wooden bases of the bed, with some light covering to them and the natural feather quilts, but not on the mattresses. I had spent some time testing these, and put the compromising affect on my pulses down to the metal springs inside the mattress.

I did not protest when rebuilding the bedroom to how we originally found it, (although I did make the passing suggestion that I could sleep on the wooden base and make up her side to how it was before) but instead apologised for sabotaging our stay and my wife's pleasure, I knew my behaviour was a little excessive. My wife wanted to enjoy the comfort we were paying for during our stay and I could not deny her this opportunity. A couple of nights spent in a luxury hotel room we had travelled half way across Europe to experience were not going to kill me. I would be doing more harm to myself no doubt through drinking and smoking, than an expensive sprung mattress could ever achieve in a couple of nights. I put my loss of perspective down to my pre-existing materials mania becoming aggravated by the long drive that day.

Part III

Evolving tests, food shopping and cooking.

Being guided in my decisions regarding clothing, bedding and shoes via the pulses works fine in private, with just my dear wife to witness these experiments and tests, but as experienced when testing out the belts in the High Street stores, it is more risky performing these tests in public places, without alerting the concerns of others, even when doing my best to remain discrete.

A particular matter I'd been dealing with was the extent that my mind has influence upon the pulses, so to help overcome any confusion this caused when testing I would perform the same test of an item several times over, with and then without the test matter, to be sure I was not imagining or unduly conjuring a false reading. The problem with this approach is that in practise it requires me to pick up, then put down, then pick up, and put down again, and possibly up and down again, whilst simultaneously holding the wrist of one hand with the other, and carefully sense what the pulses are doing. It's not very discrete in practise, and getting a reliable reading requires time and a lot of patience, and of course a calm mind. Where testing clothing is concerned in the high street I'm sure it looks like I'm just about to make a run for the doors and just look all nonchalant for the purpose of picking my best time to dash out, in maintaining the clothing article close by or in my hand.

I'd soon moved on to testing the foods in my local supermarket stores using my pulses just out of interest in what I could determine. My first observations were made in the cheaper food store, where the shelving and displays were too close together and the resultant atmosphere somewhat chaotic from the view point of keeping my mind neutral and non-thinking, and in minimising my thoughts influence on the response to my tests. Chaotic shopping environments made it much harder to be able to notice a sufficient difference between my readings to be certain of what was being experienced. I considered that some of this chaos may have been caused by the way food items were being mixed up on the shelves, with heavily processed foods being located next to those less processed food items I was more drawn towards testing. Further, the more toxic caustic items such as cleaning products were sometimes in close proximity to foodstuffs, which

I thought influenced my tests. So I preferred shopping at the nicely organised, wider aisled shopping environment of the more expensive supermarket store in my high street, in spite of us living on a bit of a budget. There were fewer hectic shoppers and the atmosphere much more peaceful an experience, helpful in my shopping with the senses. I felt it allowed me to make better choices, and fewer poor purchasing decisions from the view of my senses, so all in all it was no more expensive if one is to think about it from the sense friendly view.

However even in the higher quality shopping environs I still found it quite a challenge to hold an item, whilst pretending to read the label, putting my mind to neutral and holding the wrist of the hand holding the item to take my pulse. Whilst performing this complex manoeuvre I also had to remain alerted to the nice supermarket store security officer. I already had had a minor run in with him, concerning my preference to shop with the hessian shopping bags of the supermarket, used to take goods home in, as opposed to the metal shopping basket provided for the purpose of selecting products before check out. I had to insist to him that I was not a shoplifter and that I would continue to shop the way I chose. I apologised to him after our run in, and said that I hoped he understood that I wasn't trying to be difficult and how I appreciated he was just trying to do his job and follow company policy, (which I was flouting). I mean I couldn't really tell him I was allergic to metals, or worse that my senses didn't like the baskets, that might have sounded too suspect for him, and I'm risking a ban from my favourite supermarket here, for literally being a basket case. Thereafter I always made a point to say hello and wish him well whenever I visited the store, in the hope I could pacify any remnant concerns in him about my dubious shopping habits.

Within my practice as a therapist and acupuncturist, now without needles, for some time I had been trying to teach and focus upon breathing techniques with every patient, after reading about how important it was to breath into the lower abdomen, using the diaphragm, to benefit the patient. In the beginning of this breathing phase of mine, in introducing breathing techniques to my clients, I had to somehow reconcile the aim of my therapy with myself. Whilst patients would be seeking assistance for nothing related to the breath in their own view, would it not seem strange to them that I was spinning their treatment dollar and time by teaching and encouraging them in how to breath for occasionally more than just a few minutes at the start of a treatment? To be honest back then I could not really make the connection between therapy and breathing for myself in a plausible

Shaun M Sutton

way but maintained the teaching of breathing, for the sake of interest and feeling there likely was something in it.

In my endeavours to help patients to breath better, I would ask them if they knew where their diaphragm muscle was located and try to help them appreciate what happens on their inside for a breath to occur. I even had a syringe on my equipment trolley to demonstrate the visual analogy of a breath, pulling the plunger down to show diaphragmic inhalation, and pushing the plunger up for exhalation, and forcing the air out. (See appendices 2, 3 and 4 for further details upon diaphragmic breathing)

More recently I have been dipping in and out of the translations of a few ancient Chinese philosophy texts, such the Chuang Tzu, Tao Te Ching and a work of Ko Hung's, in which all make comments at some point on the importance of breathing for the health and well-being of the human condition, tied into some deep or mystical philosophical thought. At the time though, whilst of course Yoga too places great importance on the breath, actually tying it in with therapy work for conditions unrelated to the breath continued to feel a bit weak to me and beyond the comprehension of some of my patients.

Yet through persistence in encouraging diaphragmic breathing, I did begin to note that after a good responsive treatment a patient's breathing into the low abdomen looked easier and more comfortable. This was as opposed to them breathing more with the chest, which is how they had often began in the session.

About the time of my pulse testing of all things, I read an article in an acupuncture journal I subscribe, the North American Journal of Oriental Medicine (NAJOM) in the July 2009 issue. An acupuncture and Shiatsu practitioner with over 30 years practise, Kamiya Kazunobu from Toronto, wrote an article valuable for me entitled 'Paying Attention to the Breath'. This reported that most patients who do not demonstrate the breath change also experienced less treatment effect in his observations. The author questioned just what is the connection between this breath change phenomenon and treatment effect.

So coupling my own thoughts with those of the article I began experimenting using my diaphragmic breathing as a more surreptitious testing method when out shopping, considering an improved breath to indicate a positive response, in the same way a softening and relaxing of the pulses was to me. In making the diaphragmic breathing tests whilst holding the radial pulse there existed a correlation between the relaxed nature of the pulse and ease of inhalation in trying this out on the things I was testing.

To begin with when out shopping, I could only inhale to a count of 5 or 6 in my mind when testing, the longer the count reflecting the more positive response in my own view. This initial lack of breath to work with as a response caused me to add in making observation concerning the ease of my breath, as much as its count in my mind for the time taken to inhale fully with the diaphragm.

Armed with the new response testing tool, my diaphragmic breath for measuring the material world, shopping then became a great adventure, albeit timely experience. My wife would question the length of time I spent out shopping, as I'd often be for gone a considerable amount of time. I found I had to shop alone, as we could no longer do the food shopping together. She could not help feel a little impatient with me continually stopping to test the foodstuffs, which I found a distraction for performing my tests when attempting to not think and have a neutral mind during my testing process. Instead I would end up thinking about my wife's anxieties, worried about her being hungry and annoyed with me for delaying the cooking in order to test the foods out before I purchased them. It was easier to consider the responses when shopping alone.

The most brilliant thing about testing with the breath is that it is incredibly discrete, even though at first the testing continued to make me feel somewhat guilty or sneaky, as though I should not be doing it. However this was an undercover or secret world I was trying to reveal for myself, adding a whole new dimension to the concept of a secret shopper. Now I could mill about the store holding things, inconspicuously gazing at the ingredients on the packaging labels, or just pretending to be qualified in contemplating how I could use this or that in a meal, whilst holding an item and testing it with my ease of inhalation. During my years of being a practitioner I have come across or read about many different ways to test things in some similar fashion.

My first experience of someone testing something whilst shopping was over 15 years before, during the time when I ran a skin care salon. In the first year of the business, fairly soon after we had opened, a pleasant and friendly woman who we had never seen before comes into the store, says hello and how much she liked what we were doing. She then asked if I minded her dowse test the different moisturisers to find out which one was most suited to her skin. I didn't know anything on this subject at the time, but said sure whatever you wish to do (for me to hopefully make a sale and have a happy customer). She then takes out a crystal on a chain and hovers it over a selection of different moisturisers and cleansers, allowing it to swing in its own rhythm as she tested each product. My business partner, who was doing the accounts at the time, hidden from view behind our tall reception desk, nudged my leg saying under her breath "get her out of here, she's a nutter", whilst the relaxing music provided a cover for her words. I ignored her suggestion, and let the woman work in her own time without interruption. The thing I never considered at the time was that she could have decided from her tests that she did not like any of them.

This customer, Jayne, happened to be a Reiki Master and we became good friends after, as well as she a regular customer. In fact it was through her teaching me Reiki and initiating me to the consideration that some other sort of world existed to the one I'd grown up in, that had lead me to study herbal medicine. So different was this alternative Reiki world to my old one, that for reasons of maintaining my own sanity I enrolled to study herbal medicine, hoping to hang out and hopefully study with some similarly minded potential weirdoes as myself, and to at least be able to discuss the stranger aspects of the world I seemed to be coming into contact with. I got my wish, as a number of my fellow herbal students turned out to in fact also be Reiki Masters. (Reiki is a Japanese hands on and distant healing system)

Becoming open to a whole 'other world' of possibilities in how things work is a tricky business for one's sanity, well mine at least, like there is no longer a safety net of normality to rely upon, which I had found unsettling at that time of my Reiki investigations. Maybe it's just me having a difficulty here, everyone else seemed to act either all together with themselves or be completely out there with the fairies and beyond even my own bounds. It was all a bit too far removed from my own kind of small country village mentality that I had grown up with in Sussex. In my own village definitely such things were beyond the mind of the reasonable person, and so I struggled a lot to come to terms with what could be real, from what was a mere figment of my imagination. Jayne, my Reiki Master friend had said to me, at the time of my Reiki level one training, that I would become sensitive to all sorts of stuff as a result of the Reiki training. I had become overly open to my own suggestions, I think that is the best way to put it, I was on the edge back then, far too open, before I moved on to a world more tangible to play in. Now again, with all my pulse and breath testing, I felt I was approaching upon some similar level of uncertainty about my world, however this time around I had more tools to help me out, and in particular my means to response test, that was a tangible in my eyes.

Testing things by way of the pulse and now the breath, allowed me to hopefully keep a more real and physical fix on my sensitivities to the world, as opposed to relying on my feelings, emotional sensitivities and mental conceptualisations of the more spiritual world I had so greatly struggled with in the past, as a relative novice practitioner those years before.

I began discretely testing all sorts of things in the supermarket. Was stone ground or white organic flour best for my responses? Or would it be Rye, Millet, or the ancient Spelt flour? Were organic or free range, or conventionally farmed products any different to each other? Milk, deserts, sauces, deserts, sugar, teas, beer, cider, local grown, seasonal or imported produce, fish or beef for dinner, or beans, which kind? Olive oils, is there any difference between them all perceivable with the breath?

All these questions could be now considered through quietly testing using my diaphragmic inhalation procedure, without any fear of suspicion, or being spotted in what I was doing. Much less obvious than dowsing in public, being less concern raising amongst the unknowing and potentially easily unsettled public at large, or the store security officer they may potentially send to my shopping aisle, he already knew I was one to keep an eye on. Now I had the whole store of foods in which to investigate and study in my own time without fear of being found out for what I was practising. Hopefully my wife would not get too hungry whilst I was out shopping, or that is testing for our dinner.

As a man for creating theories, I came up with several potential acronyms for this diaphragmic testing process I was working with. The first was the DIC test, being short for Diaphragmic Inhalation Capacity test, applying a schoolboy level of humour. Then next, considering the inappropriateness of talking about investigating foods with my DIC test, for my own further amusement I came up with LAPD, short for Lower Abdominal Diaphragmic Potential, which I then used for note taking as a reference for the count I made in my mind whilst inhaling for the breath capacity testing. (What about LIAR test, for lower inhalation abdominal response test?)

During these early days of testing whilst shopping, or in making selection based upon the breath capacity, several observations most stood out to me in all this. The first was that I could not test anything in a container made of any metal, this concealed my response to the contents as a result of my response to the material of the container overwhelming that of the contents. However I seemed to have no difficulty in testing items held in plastic, glass or paper packaging, with no interference for the test coming from these packaging materials. The other matter about food shopping in general is the many situations when I am unable to actually hold and touch the food or the container to test it, such as at the cold foods counter or in the genuine fresh produce stands at the more traditional markets of Germany in my own experience. In the markets it seemed to me impossible or inappropriate for me to go around touching foods on display without actually buying what I touched, or the food items I wanted were located out of reach behind the staff at the market stalls. So I could not test everything before buying, but maybe this is just a cultural issue of some form.

Where buying meats was concerned in the supermarket I could test the pre-packed items, and then go to the cold counter and ask for what I then considered was testing well for me that day. This way the article was potentially fresher, and it saved on environmental landfill from packaging waste. The fact that the meats were raw and uncooked did not seem to prove a problem in my tests, especially for something like chicken. Even so I don't think I would be prepared to trust my senses so well as to then try eat the chicken raw.

One weekend I lined up 'the big blind egg test', involving four different types of chicken eggs, from cage reared to free range, and organic. I had accidentally purchased, on good faith (as I had not been able to test them at the time of purchase), a dozen of what turned out to be barn laid eggs from the Saturday French cheese man in his van, having assumed that he would only take the trouble in bringing some sort of super exotic farm egg all the way from France along with his famed fine quality unpasturised cheeses. So I was surprised when getting the eggs home to discover, on translating the label my worst fears, 'cage or barn reared', which is almost the same thing to me. This highlights the problem of buying over a counter on trust, plus how we are so easily duped into buying something that we think is authentic on appearance, only to later uncover flaws in what it does for us if maybe tested against the responses. This later point is the most important of all matters associated with buying anything for me, so many things look like the real thing but on comparative response testing they certainly are not the authentic article, making them in some way just fake.

On initially testing the cage barn eggs I had felt they hardened my pulses and reduced the diaphragmic inhalation capacity, so I gave a half dozen of these cage barn eggs to a neighbour, who couldn't really understand why I didn't want them but accepted them anyway. The remainder I kept for the big blind egg test.

On the outside an egg is an egg, but could I tell the difference between the means each had been produced through just my own application of the senses and responses? I thought it a good test, but basically the test ended up as inconclusive and perhaps I'd involved my mind in some way, thinking oh this must be the cage egg, and this the corner shop organic, and that one organic from the supermarket, as in the end the French barn cage reared egg now came out as OK compared with the others according to the responses. Maybe it was OK, but even so I didn't eat the cage eggs out of principle, that's the power of negative marketing. This was a reminder that maybe my tests were flawed and useless and I, a sad, delusional and misguided individual who really should get on with more important things in his life than messing about wasting his time testing everything. I had to consider this as a possibility, that I could be a little 'off the boil'.

Then came cooking, I did the majority of cooking at home, as a modern man the kitchen has always been my domain and not my wife's, which was a big help for testing and deciding what to eat according to my own breath and pulse. Once the food is prepared it's a bit late for testing, so my idea was to test the ingredients as I assembled them for the pot, not using anything that was less positive than neutral upon the breath and pulse. This seemed to work out, and it proved a useful exercise to re-test the items I had previously tested at the time of purchase. It was often the case that I found something having previously tested fine did no longer and visa versa. Food articles I had thought of as having been response mistaken purchases often again turned out as agreeable to the responses. Patterns of response were inconsistent, indicating that either my tests were not working, or that my taste needs were changing. However, at that time salty and foods with vinegar or sugar added in them always tested out badly, the likes of ketchup a no-no, so these food stuffs and especially condiments, were left out of the cooking. However my wife likes the salty and vinegar foods so she just added whatever she wanted to the meal according to her own tastes at the time of serving. That way neither of us needed to compromise on our needs.

Shaun M Sutton

I do feel that food preparation and selection, if performed according to the senses, is a potential minefield in a family environment, but hey maybe that's been a contributor to why the world ended up leaving the senses redundant for serving our needs, especially where the person doing the cooking is not the one using their senses to find their own preferences. In our home situation it worked out convenient with just the two of us. Maybe this sort of approach to cooking would work out in the family setting, I've never tested it, but it may possibly involve the diners eating from a variety of dishes as opposed to everyone eating the same thing as we tend towards in our Western culture.

After many shopping expeditions and attempts at food preparation according to my breath and pulse responses, I developed a fairly good feel for what was likely to be at least neutral in effect, and knew that certain commonly used foods and ingredients in foods were definitely to be avoided by me from a response view, after repeated tests had been confirming the same compromise to the responses. As a result I was able to spend less time testing and shopping, saving the tests for when I thought I should double check something, rather than just make theoretically based decision. This freed me up for the other more important things I needed to get on with. You need time to test things with the responses. I admit to it being a bit of a bind I probably did not really have the time for in the beginning

Once a food dish is prepared you have to eat it, that's been my rule, otherwise this testing thing is really making life far too complicated and difficult. I even had a suspicion that the hungrier one is, the greater the variety of foods one will have a positive test response to and the more things one could eat without getting a negative response. I have however found that even with all the best selection means and intentions possible for ingredients, meals sometimes ended up with me feeling bloated, whacked out and tired, or kept me awake at night due to the 'eat it if you've cooked it' rule, or something else I was unaware of.

What is harder to work out is the point where sufficient has been eaten to satisfy the responses and to not overeat, and to become aware of how the cooking process influences the responses to the food, so monitoring my failed meals as far as how I generally felt after helped some in this. Occasionally I would not eat a meal but this is where someone else had prepared it other than me. Eating out was more often a dreadful experience where the responses were concerned, but I live in England on a budget so I hear you say, "what do you expect!". (I don't think the food in England is quite as bad as the press it is sometimes given) In fact I would go as far as to say that eating out in general was only occasionally a positive experience for my responses, but when it was that has been a wonderful thing.

I am really stunned that we can all live as we do, evolution is an incredible thing, man has evolved to be able to feed himself with foods our senses perhaps would hands down reject, that is truly amazing. Equally over the years I have read and heard such an incredible variety of nutritional theories from doctors, experts and the like, each providing the ultimate way to feed ourselves, without using the senses, that it makes me wonder how it all works, or I think that is 'how we work'. Then we have regulations to protect us from ourselves, but these same regulations risk limiting our freedom of choice. Take the case of cheese and pasteurisation, me I want the choice to have cheese from raw milk if I wish. The French cheese man in the van says it really is considered as better for us. Maybe it is, or maybe is his own brand of marketing to sell us his cheese. But raw milk products have had a rough ride of it for a while and still do in some places like in the USA, at least that is how it seemed from during my last visit.

The thing is I'm fed up of blindly, or even being forced into, following what other people advise or instruct me on as being the correct to do, but I still didn't really quite know what it is I was working with here with my testing. Is this just my own issues with authority I ask myself? This is a tricky point, but could it be that I can use the breath and pulse to not just tell me more about my trousers and clothing, or what I should and should not eat, but also to guide me in the best way to lead my life some how? In the absence of an appropriate teacher in such things it really came down to me acting as my own guide if I wanted to have a go at working it out. It seemed like I didn't have much choice in the matter, of course I was interested in working it out, having gone so far there was no apparent reason to turn back, or revert back to the world as we currently know it, and I had known it.

In the mornings that Autumn I would go into the garden at the back of my home and exercise. Over several weeks I observed the English garden Blackbirds gobbling down the red and orange berries off the shrubbery, and should any other bird go near, they would chase them off, vigilantly defending their territory's berry crop. Next to these berry heavy shrubs were growing some Deadly Nightshade, itself also covered in red berries the same size as the other berries, but the Blackbirds were not eating these, whether they could do I don't know I'm no expert in birds.

I'd never given thought to this matter before, of how these birds knew what to eat and what not to, without trial and error poisonings occurring. Maybe the foxes ate those birds self-poisoned during the night, as there was no sign of them the next day. Or could it be there is something in us too, a wild side, that could allow us to know, like the Blackbird, what to eat, when to stop, and was it this that I was beginning to work with, my wild side? Is there some sort of ancient part of me that had not in reality become lost during human evolution and centuries of incredible change in how we live? I reckoned this was most likely what I had been attempting to rekindle and tap into without realising, my own essence of the wild.

Part IV

Testing clothing and other materials

Whilst shopping with the guidance of my breath, I regularly found it difficult to disseminate my responses to what I was attempting to assess, in helping decide what I should or should not purchase. I experienced difficulty concentrating during the test in environments not naturally encouraging to inhalation using the diaphragm, either as a result of the nature of the shopping environment, or how I was feeling on the day. It was all a bit up and down.

I began to notice other responses in myself beyond the breath and pulse when testing, the most common being for a negative response by way of a tightening or stiffening sensation in the chest and neck muscles. Whilst trying to remain as neutral in my mind as possible when testing, general emotions or images and thoughts conjured by or associated with the item being tested were often a trouble to bypass. I put this down to the influence of the environment I was in or as a general negative response.

Some days, when I'd had a more easy going and relaxing day, finding the neutral mind state, allowing me to just focus on doing the tests, was a much easier and quicker an affair. There were certain things that always proved to be consistently negative in my responses, which then provided me a negative response bench mark to compare my responses to other things being tested. The genuine negative responses reminded me there was something to all this after all, and think, ah that feels better when testing and comparing it to something more positive. This was a bit of a lifeline to reality, feeling a known negative response during those earlier days when I was less certain of these testing ideas. Certain of these negative response items and things were a surprise to me because so many of them I had used regularly in the past. What affect had these been having on me over all these years? It could explain a lot about me and perhaps even help explain away some of my less than pleasant life events and past behaviour.

Patience was a necessary requirement in testing, without applying it I easily made severe errors of judgement of my responses, especially under those less than favourable shopping environments, to end up purchasing things I later found were leading to poor breath and response. In fact I could say that if I lacked sufficient patience to double or triple check my responses to something and wanted to make a snap decision, then there was a very high likelihood it would give a negative response later, and I was just kidding myself into believing it was ok. There was definitely a pattern emerging along such lines. Observing my own levels of patience was interesting because I have previously had an impetuous character.

There were always a lot of my own questions. "Was a previous response just a one off as a result of me having a bad test day, flawed by impatience and misread response?" There was also the matter of doing too much testing, which reduced my ability to test, so some days I would literally just have to call it a day and know when I was beat, get away and sort myself out, come back to it another day. This was sometimes harder to do than it sounds, and if I kept going I would make poor reading of my LAPD or DIC. If I'd set it in my mind I wanted something I'd have difficulty in stopping and holding myself back from a poor judgement call of the responses. This was a battle between the will of my mind against my senses and responses in controlling my purchasing decisions.

A crucial development came when I began going clothes shopping with the breath for guidance during my frequent visits to a bunch of wonderful second hand clothing stores near my home. I now loved shopping for clothes, like a child looking for toys to buy. I'd never realised clothes shopping or buying second hand clothes could be so interesting until I began to observe my responses could be so different to different fabrics, a revelation. This I found to be a relaxing past-time to pursue, and if I had an hour spare or going that way home, I would pop in to see what was there, going from one charity shop to the next looking at the second hand clothes.

Nobody cares if you linger at a second hand item of clothing, or holding it, it is what normal people do, and so I could feel more relaxed and patient in my testing. In new clothing stores I could not do this, there should be no reason to do this in these stores really, to fondle and inspect the clothing, and then you have the sales assistants paid to help, or hound, and keep an eye on you. The second hand clothing shops allowed me certain extra liberties beneficial for my response testing of the materials the clothes were made up of and allow me the time and space to really go to town on my testing to find a truly wonderful item on the racks. This is what made clothes shopping so exciting and enjoyable to me, it was like a game or test, could I spot the genuine article from the impostor, by way of just using my responses and senses?

I began ruling out certain fabrics and materials as being unsuitable for a positive response, mostly these were synthetic fibres but not always, several natural materials too proving unsuitable, which was a surprise and had caught me out because at times I shopped like anyone else, with my head and not my senses. I had to smarten up my means of selecting potential purchases otherwise I ended up returning things I'd just bought the other day, and without any refund possibility given in these shops.

Whilst not all synthetic fibres were a problem, materials made from blends of natural mixed with unfavourable synthetic fibres were a challenge to ascertain response, in that one small part would provide a negative response. But in the end I went purist as I found that my senses got very confused with these blends, like my body was having problems working it out with the responses. Even if there was just 5 or 10% of a negative response material in something, I believed I could sense my response to this, but it was definitely harder to pick it up sometimes, especially when it was quite a nice item or something I had been looking for and I'm considering the garment's other positive attributes for myself. Higher proportions than 20% or so negative response material were generally not too hard to spot. The labels helped in this learning and educational testing process I was going with.

Sometimes I had some hard decisions to make as a result of finding a clothing article made of all the right things for me, even fitting reasonably, but colour wise was on the edge of, or beyond what I previously considered as acceptable and tasteful. In the end after a few blatant errors of my judgement and some crazy styles or colours, I agreed with my wife to not wear these articles in public places, or at least not when with her. Thereafter I would have the girls in the charity shops put the item aside for my wife to double check later with me, which overcame my over zealous enthusiasm when finding that something I had been looking for. I saw the positive in this, and not that I was being efficiently quality controlled by my German spouse.

The only thing I was unable to test were the women's clothes, which took up the greater floor area in these second hand clothing stores. I was occasionally tempted and had made a few quick tests, but knew this would not be so easy to explain away, so I have been limited to the world of men's clothing. I have not been trying out my wife's clothes, but like to inspect the labels of her own clothing purchase decisions and pass on my potentially groundless observations.

Another matter of great fascination was in how many of the design labels had the tendency to incorporate the use of blends and integrate certain materials I responded negatively to within a great number of their articles, myself noting which labels commonly used those materials. This created a whole educational world for myself of the clothing manufacture industry, a great insight into how each brand appeared to operate in order to make a profit, and the basis behind their strategy for carving themselves a place in the fashion market.

It wasn't just the case of who the manufacturers were, but also where and how many years ago an article was made, giving me a feel to the history behind all this. Incorporation of these more modern fibres, the one's I was not responding well to, appears to be a rather recent trend as the older articles did not much include them. Also the materials I felt compromising of my responses were generally, but not always, being used in the garments produced more cheaply in the distant lands of the East. Going second hand clothes shopping with the breath as guide was like doing a graduate foundation clothing and fashion course, studying the trends and ways of clothing manufacturers and design brands.

Along with certain fabrics coming up as a definite no-no for me, so too did certain brand labels, knowing what they tended to include concerning my responses.

Shaun M Sutton

I also began excluding garments made in certain countries, not because of reasons such as the potential for sweat shop labour or that they were commonly prone to using materials my responses were unhappy with, but they often looked terrible on their hangers after what appeared to be a relatively short period of use from new (I was very fussy for a second hand clothing shopper). I have to ask, why? Why does it seem to me that so many things are now made that just don't last, is it just a matter of needs or tastes not lasting or are we, the consumer, plain ignorant or something else? Is it that in reality people are not sufficiently refined to notice the differences between what is on offer? Maybe the refined look is a fashion statement in itself, which all consumers are not into following I could guess, just thinking of several of the fashion orientated gangs out there, which seem revel about living out of these late 20th century toxic fibres, as far as my own responses seemed to be concerned.

The high street clothing stores commonly seemed to be in the habit of selling a lot of rubbish as far as I could test with my responses, and by the way many of their articles ended up looking like on the hangers of the second hand clothing stores. Yet there is a market for it as far as is visible, the system many manufacturers work with must be forcing them to cut corners, potentially achieving cost savings or functional gain, by way of introducing materials I was experiencing my toxic response to within the blends or the linings, or even just a part of the linings. I'm certain no one involved is aware that by making such savings they are potentially negatively influencing the responses of their consumers, consumers for whom the item is being designed and paid for by, and most likely have no idea to any potential for consequence upon their responses. So does it just come down to the basic matters of price, fashion and functionality being the more important matters in the manufacture? Life of use for the item seems to have lost importance, by the look of things to some significant extent, particularly in consideration of the quality of the materials being currently used. The industry as a whole appears to not be sustainable the way it is on many levels. From a production and marketing strategy view it appears as though clothing made cheaply and using materials, that I guess are cheaper yet unfriendly to my own responses, are being dump marketed, undercutting prices, and during economically difficult times the consumer is falling for the strategy, leading those producing the better quality items, I personally seek, to work within whichever niche market they can carve out for themselves, which to me appears to generally materialise as selling less volume at a higher price tag strategy. I'm guessing this is common knowledge within the Industry, and I have not the experience nor figures to support this.

I have noticed it is becoming more difficult recently to find much decent men's clothing in the second hand shops, but that might be because of reasons other than there being a reduced demand for the new quality items my senses and responses are looking for. The quality items I seek, according to my responses to their materials and likely life of use, do seem to be becoming generally harder to find, especially when shopping on a budget. Should the size of our pockets become the factor determining the materials used to make our clothing? I guess so, but is it that if we are poor we are being forced to wear toxic? I guess this is not much different a situation to that of purchasing many things. Where clothing is concerned you just need to take a look at what's on the hangers in my local charity shops to see what I mean with the quality of once new articles, how they are is not my personal cup of tea simply due to the reasons I have been describing. And yet, hands up, I admit that up until fairly recently to have been someone previously dressing myself in a lot of the fabrics and labels I was now rejecting on the men's hangers. But back then I had not been aware of any problem, I don't think I was making any fashion or other statement through wearing clothes made in those materials I was now deeming as unfriendly to my responses. They were just clothes, like that's just food, or that's just a bed, and I didn't back then give it any more thought. Had I always been this way, my clothes toxic to my responses and I just didn't know it, or is it that I, or the world, had somehow changed, or my responses have adapted to a changed world in some way?

If for arguments sake we could say that everyone is responding in the same way as I am to our everyday materials, then what does this indicate? If this is actually so, we are being duped into buying these articles for the sake of someone making a buck or two extra out of us, or we the consumer are duping ourselves for the sake of saving a buck or two, or the designers and manufacturers are duping the buyers by undercutting supply costs to get the contract by cutting back on quality through making material substitutions. Which ever way one looks at it, perhaps all are duping each other or are simply allowing themselves to be duped through a lack of knowledge on the effect upon them of the different fabrics, as far as I have been observing by my senses and responses, although the labels do after all tell us what the item is made of and the country of manufacture. Is it just that in general we have not yet gotten around to working out what the labels potentially suggest in terms of our responses, or how long the item will serve our needs. Is this simply a matter to be resolved through the purchasers getting around to using their senses, and as such generating a market with these in consideration?

We could now almost have a situation, which appears to me to be the case, where our purchasing opportunities as consumers are being so squeezed towards these junk items I am referring to, being those I would not buy myself even second hand, that the choice to buy a better quality item is not so readily available anymore, and where available the better quality article has become relatively even more expensive? It almost appears as though we have been living in a junk mentality toxic throw away era for so long we generally have less understanding of what quality is anymore. From what I can see, the older clothing items are made of generally better quality materials, as far as my own responses are concerned, and look good many years after they were made, as viewed on the second hand clothing rails. These are the 'Vintage' items now. Maybe I'm wrong, I am no fashion designer, and not really much of a consumer either, but have we been living in an era where our senses are being undermined by the materials we are using, maybe even every hour in every day.everyday? It's nothing new, being tricked to believe something is what it isn't, with items made to look and feel like something else, imitations of the real thing. This is human nature one is up against, there has always been the 'fake' about to dupe the unwitting or uneducated in such things and simply there are those who desire to fool the rest of the world.

Some years ago, way before this time of pulse and breath, I won a week long trip to go to an international skin care congress in Hong Kong, for myself with several work colleagues. Whilst there, the girls I travelled with dragged me along on an adventure, going just across the border into mainland China, to visit this dreadful shopping centre in search of counterfeit Louis Vuitton hand bags or Prada, I'm not sure which, maybe both. Pulled out from above the ceiling tiles in refuse bin liners were the sought after bags as I observed, me following from one vendor to another, the girls trying to find the most authentic looking counterfeit. It was quite an education to see how many different counterfeit qualities existed, whilst the girls coarsely haggled over the prices of their booty. Everything there you needed to haggle upon over the price, it was an irritating kind of sport where no one could have a conscience. But maybe our ignorance as consumers, on what quality really means, has allowed some level of overflow of the trading principles from the black market into the mainstream markets, and encouraging such a great penetration of the fabrics I am personally questioning into our society's wardrobes. As consumers are concerned, I vouch for us being on the whole pretty ignorant in these matters, so we cannot but help purchase what is available. Wearing any materials toxic to us has to, to some extent, prevent us using our senses, and so in a way these materials would keep us blind and in the dark to what is really going on here, a denudation of the senses as a result of what we wear.

Investigating all my clothes at home lead me to really began to clear up my own wardrobe in line with my responses, disposing of even more clothing, things I had hung onto during my anti-metals period, even clearing out a few recent purchases with unfavourable inclusions within their material construction. In fact I was left with hardly any clothes remaining at all. What a great way to make space, if it's not agreeable with the responses it has to go. I was going to the second hand charity clothing stores with bags of clothing no longer fit for my responses and coming home with a very few carefully selected items I was proud of and happy to wear, and my inhalation capacity began to grow along with it. Now my journey with the responses was just beginning.

As mentioned our funds were very limited, so each purchase had to be good and considered according to necessity. For me having a response friendly wardrobe was a necessity, my wife may have at times thought otherwise so this was some sort of role reversal we had going on. I really wanted a proper pair of all leather upper and soled shoes, the converted Redwing boots I continued living out of were better than rubber soled, but still not completely 100% earthing on natural surfaces. A customer of mine had a pair of Chelsea Boots I admired, all leather upper and sole, no metal, and instead with elasticated sides to allow squeezing the foot in and holding the boot on. We found some made in the UK on the Internet at a good price, and I admit to asking my Mum to get them for me, and I would pay her back. They seemed acceptable, but made my foot a bit sore at my right big toe and whilst they looked good they did not feel entirely right somehow. My second disappointing shoe purchase decision. (Although I must say the company I dealt with managed the complaint to my satisfaction)

Then whilst out trawling the charity shops, soon after buying my new leather Chelsea boots, I somehow picked up that my responses did not like Elastin, also referred to as Lycra. Everyone wears it, perhaps there is not one single person in this day's developed world that goes without it, except me maybe, although it is a bit inconvenient living without it to be honest. So, the Chelsea all leather boots purchase was now a complete failure for me, as now I don't wear anything that contains Elastin or Lycra, or Spandex, it has many names and yet its made of the same stuff, used to keep things up, and the boots were loaded with it by way of their elastication. I remember in the old days we had latex rubber elastic for this purpose and how after a while it would perish and go all gooey, and the clothing saggy, which Elastin has overcome it appears, so it really is a shame that my responses didn't like it.

The other thing necessary to complete the response friendly outfit was to cut out all of the labels from my clothes. I found that even in completely natural and good quality clothing, the label is in general made from cheap synthetic material, except for in a few better quality designer wear items. As far as I was concerned, even a small amount of a compromising material near or against my skin can be distinguished by the senses, which indicates it is compromising to the senses and responses, but the situation with labels is as with fabric blends, because the quantity used is small and so it is more confusing for the responses to observe.

Now I was really able to confidently go about doing all my shopping in completely, or as close to as I could sense, a response friendly outfit. Anything less than completely response friendly had now been mostly ruled out of my life at each opportunity availing me, even where alternatives were not available. I began with shopping in my old leather soled Redwing boots, then I found a second hand pair of all leather upper and sole shoes for a bargain price. With all wool socks, response friendly attire, no belt, no underpants, yes because of the Elastin, and now no synthetic care labels, I was better equipped and able to spot any inferior materials in clothing items as a result. This seemed to lead to a further increase in my lower abdominal inhalation capacity, and to a greater degree of sensitivity to detect those materials I was seeking to avoid through just observing my breath. Due to the longer count, in the LAPD, it was easier to recognise anything unfavourable to my responses. My inhalation count jumped to 11 or so when generally out and about.

These jumps have been kind of ongoing. Now when I'm in a really good way I inhale with my diaphragm to a count of between 35 and 50, which in a way could be a good thing on one level, but on the other hand it now takes much longer to test something, although testing is now more accurate. This could be the result of the diaphragm muscle strengthening on account of all the diaphragmic breathing I was doing, or something else, but really this just indicates where I was then as compared with at the time of writing concerning my breathing. The main thing to appreciate now is that differences in response became much more obvious as my scale of testing enlarged, through my breath, leading to generally more accurate decisions from my breath capacity tests of things around me. (refer to the appendices 2, 3 and 4 for more in depth information on testing with the breath)

As a part of purging all response unfriendly materials from my life, where ever convenient, our bed continued to evolve, along with my sleeping habits. I disposed of all my bedding, the duvet quilt and pillows, unfriendly upon my responses, but I had nothing to replace them with. My wife was not ready to make the same shift. To be honest I think that her holding onto these articles of bedding was her way of holding onto some sort of normality considering all the changes I was making, plus and more importantly, she was not prepared to sleep like a tramp in her own bed as I was. I respected this, so I let her sleep on her side of the new natural futon with the remainder of the bedding, now unsuitable for me, in her pyjamas, and I slept on my side using a couple of rolled up towels to make a pillow for my head, in a T shirt inside a big heavy Bolivian wool jumper with multi-coloured cats knitted into it from the charity shop, and basically nothing else other than real wool socks, since my pyjamas have an Elastin waist band to them, and so I would not wear them. I then used a few big towels to cover me for sleeping. We could not afford that final major financial investment necessary to completely upgrade our bedding to the response friendly standard I was looking for.

In spite of feeling like I was sleeping rough, I hold fond memory of this time, it was liberating, like sleeping in the woods but with more comfort. I was taking complete control of my environment, as much as our means allowed. On the down side I developed a phobia to my wife's side of the bed due to the old toxic bedding she was maintaining. When going to bed I would make sure her quilt was well over her side so that I should not become contaminated during my sleep, by way of either of us accidentally rolling to the other's side. I think that it sounds worse than it was in practice, many couples resort to separate beds after all.

Then we splashed out on a couple of good value wool filled pillows from the same place we had purchased the futon, and I had a complete stroke of luck in one of the second hand charity stores, coming across four unused Jaipur quilts, they still had their original hand written size labels stuck on them. Up until then I had been looking at these expensive German natural fibre filled quilts, and wondering if we could ever afford them, whilst questioning how long I could continue sleeping rough like a tramp in the winter. So the Jaipur quilts were like pennies dropped from heaven, saving us and perhaps even our relationship.

These beautifully decorated quilts, the outer being in a decorative print, come from Rajistan in North West India. They were very thin and looked like they would not keep us warm at all, in comparison to the heavy regular quilts, but quite surprisingly they were great. Apparently the quilts are famous for their warmth and light weight, being used by desert nomads. Filled with special carded cotton they provided both light weight and warmth. Hey, you just learn something new every day. (Yet I must add, sometimes they may be filled with the inclusion of natural fibres that are not completely response friendly, that is from my own view, but still these are superior according the my responses as compared to certain other fibres commonly used in bedding.)

Life changing, that's what it was. It was like moving to live in a palace, no more dodgy old towels to sleep under or as my pillow, no more toxic bedding. I began sleeping without anything at all on, and I encouraged my wife to do the same and to discard, finally giving up her beloved pyjamas at night. This was on account of my next discovery, which on making now makes me extremely wary of coming up with any more theories for anything ever again. Perhaps 'suspicion' would be a more appropriate word for me to use than 'theory' in these cases.

I was lying in the new toxic-free bed, with my foot out of the side on the wood floor, as had been my habit to earth myself and I counted my LAPD, my inhalation, then snuggled my foot under the covers as it was a bit chilly, performed again the count and found that there was in fact no difference between foot out touching the floor and foot in under the warmth of the new non-toxic bed covers. This was in spite of my consideration that our futon was not completely earthing, by way of the incorporation of cotton within component layers, cotton being in my mind a semi-insulator or semi-earthing material. It seemed that all my earthing and insulators, earthing pathways terminology and theory I'd been using for myself just no longer mattered, was irrelevant, redundant on some level in how I had to now view the world according to the way my body was responding to my environment.

It appeared that on some level there is no response to the beneficial effects of earthing when one is in an environment without the influence of anything that is response unfriendly, i.e., a totally response friendly environment, or so it seemed. All my ideas had to be adjusted as a result of this observation. Earthing theory was to be shelved for now, its place less significant. I still prefer barefoot, leather soles, wool socks, and natural surfaces to walk upon, but am now a bit happier wearing rubber soled boots for practical reasons, that is if everything else I wear is good for the responses.

However, in changing ideas upon how and what I orientated decision making around in my environment, and letting go of something I had been living according to the principles of, even if this was by my own theory or 'suspicion' of the response benefits of earthing materials, I am returned back to the uncertain place again. All I'm looking for is something to be navigated by according to my own instruction. Letting go of old ideas, raison d'être, theories of guidance, particularly in my professional practise, does seem to have also been a general theme for the way of things during my response testing period time right up until now. I was regularly being tested to drop my ideas, letting them go, like leaves dropping from a tree in Autumn I guess, moving on to explore some other ideas to help suit my new position and view. The basis of letting go was through considering things I was working with from a more response based view and less according to theoretical based decisions, generating a re-designing in all aspects of the way and means I worked or lived my life by.

On some level this was a kind of nightmare I found myself living in, a world made up of materials everywhere limiting my ability to apply the senses of discrimination beyond the standard theoretical choices available. A world where everyone has become reliant upon the sense free systems we have to dictate how things are and should be, a world organised to be safe to operate in, perhaps for when we cannot sense. Has man become not just blind to his own potential by way of the systems we have in place to operate under, but also a bit too comfortable with how we have it so that it's difficult to change? Would a more sense and response orientated world become an unworkably chaotic and unsafe environment, and hence the reason why we have evolved such as we have?

I asked myself how long our living environment and ways had been the way I was finding. When in Germany I was told about the Shoe Museum in Offenbach, just outside Frankfurt. I was interested to learn of how the shoe has evolved over the years and when the plastic or rubber sole had come into being. Quite recently appeared to be the case, in the fashion shoe of the 1930's, at least that is how it seemed according to the displays of shoes throughout the ages. It's only been since the 1960's or 1970's really that so much unnatural things, from foods to materials, have begun to be so heavily incorporated into how we live. But man's had his problems way before the rubber shoe sole or man made fibre revolutions, in fact we've always had problems if one comes to think about it, considering world wars and the like.

Shaun M Sutton

Was this some sort of gradual encroachment into our world by way of the synthetic materials and products that did not agree with our responses, something happening all so slowly that nobody recognised what was going on? Were we merely allowing ourselves the benefits of our technological improvements to life, of which there exist so many, or is there something else that's going on here? Is it that we are gradually poisoning ourselves without realising, and leading us further down the path of potential self destruction? Perhaps that is a tad over dramatic.

How many times has man discovered a chemical in regular use that is in fact harmful to health? How often has this lead to a kind of panic as a result? I remembered back to the Alar scare of the 1980's in the UK. Alar was applied to apples in the orchards to make their fruit redden, from memory as a kind of fruit ripener. At the time of it being banned, due to concerns over the risks being publicised, many people stopped eating apples altogether causing the apple markets to fall apart and a period of financial hardship to those producing apples due to a certain level of panic and hysteria from consumers. So what if it is actually promoted to the mass markets, in the same way of the Alar scare, that the fabrics and materials I am finding issue with, according to my responses, also are affecting other people? Would manufacturers have problems selling the now deemed toxic stocks, and what about supplying non-toxic replacements? Profits would fall, some businesses sailing too close to a margin of liquidity would fold, the people involved would loose their jobs and suffer financial hardship. Add in the fact that companies plan ahead on their next season's collections, where would that leave them if their consumers suddenly deemed the materials used in producing these collections as now being too toxic?

The question becomes, 'if we used our senses of response more, could we act before there is a problem and without any ensuing chaos or panic, could we identify the materials offending the senses and responses for ourselves?' The problem is everyone, at least in my neck of the world in London, is so incredibly busy in work and home that our society has to almost run on automatic pilot. They've hardly time to eat properly according to basic nutritional health theory, let alone mess about testing their world with responses to predict what they will respond best to in life or to prevent future catastrophe of their businesses currently supplying sense and response unfriendly products.

So, could it be mankind is destined to live in some kind of desperate loop, a noose of our own creation, keeping us reliant upon what we are told and informed of by our world, whether it's marketing or scientific research or Government regulation to make up for our lack of time and ability to check things out for ourselves? Above all else, staring at me is why to make a change, do we know what the benefit is of making any change toward a world more geared and educated to work with our senses of response?

A few years ago I tried reading some of Charles Darwin's diaries. Being written in an older, more formal, even stonier style of English they were a little beyond my regular reading range, but I came across an interesting story from his days as a Geologist, before he came up with those theories on the evolution of species.

Quoting from Darwin's Letters, Volume I, Darwin tells a story of examining a valley in Bangor Wales, in which the arrangement of rocks made no sense to him whatsoever until someone a few years after came up with all the theories of glacial movement and phenomena, which then became generally understood and accepted by the scientific community of the day. Then the way the rocks were viewed in the valley could now make complete sense from glacial theory. Darwin writes

"On this tour I had a striking instance of how easy it is to overlook phenomena, however conspicuous, before they have been observed by anyone. After I declared these phenomena as so conspicuous that in a magazine I said, a house burnt down by fire did not tell its story more plainly than did this valley"

The question really is to me, "is this just me?," plus, "would working with the senses just prove too difficult for other people to achieve, and so it's not possible to change as a society, even if we liked?" Then the other concern is that we are all different, and what works for each of us is perhaps different too, which certainly is the case in some respects. Or "are there simply too many things that we take for granted as being fine for us, that no body should actually be using if one wishes to respect the senses and responses?"

It's all well and good having fancy theories, or 'suspicions', but if no one else can see what you can then there's no point to the theory, other than for reasons of one's own amusement.

Part V

Design, Germany and my responses

My wife studied Industrial Design for 7 years at University in Germany and so this provides me with more idea about design than the average person on the street. In the same way a man buying himself some power tools cannot describe himself as a tradesman, I say I know very little about Design, and am a cowboy in these matters if saying anything different. My knowledge of Design extends as far as having hung out or got drunk with a few of my wife's designer buddies during our regularly visits to Frankfurt.

Whilst in Frankfurt, away from my work in London, I had plenty of time for testing items, perhaps even too much time on my hands. What is it they say about idle hands? Well, I had found a whole new world in which to play whilst away, the Frankfurt apartments of our generous German friends, and by way of our other experiences in Germany. I tested everything I could think of with breath and pulse responses. Because of my wife's connection to Design, I might have given a greater focus on that profession and industry than would otherwise have been the case.

I feel I appear a bit ungrateful in rewarding our generous friends with the earlier comments about their sleeping set up, so whilst at it I might as well get my money's worth and also mention how there was this long low voltage metal design lamp in their apartment, extending the full length of the dining table and hung down from the high ceiling to about 2 or 3 feet (60-90cm) from my head when seated at the table to eat, relax and chat. I can't say I could easily do so, being too concerned about my responses to the lamp. It tested that I could sense a compromising response to this lamp up to a distance of about 5 feet (1.5m). I used to sit in a child's wooden high chair instead of at the table's bench, so I could sit as far back from the lamp as was reasonable.

On the upside, in all the various apartments we were staying at, natural or wooden floors were the norm, which for me was perhaps the most essential and important of matters.

I stopped using my lap top when it was charging on the mains lead, as I felt this caused to a noticeably negative response upon the breath and pulse tests, as well as finding the titanium cased Apple Mac computer influencing my responses noticeably less detrimentally than did my old Dell equivalent laptop. So I stopped using the Dell, especially as its battery had died and it only worked off the mains lead.

I loved the choice and variety of foods available at the traditional weekly outdoor markets of Frankfurt. What a pleasant relief from England where it's all supermarkets other than a few exceptions and expensive farmers markets. At the German markets we would go and do most of the weekly shopping for bread, fruit and veg to meats, and what an incredible selection of fresh and cured meats, not forgetting the famous German sausages, the wurst. In our local Bornheim street market the quality of what was on offer was fantastic, and authentic. The problem for me was that in spite of the best quality wurst, perhaps in the world, my responses did not like any of them. We put this down to either too much salt and, or the inclusion of preservative, which was, it appeared, ladled out into everything of pre-prepared nature.

Living in Germany was actually now less healthy with the foods than I had previously appreciated. Yet a great many people, especially those of the older generation, would queue outside in the wind, rain, frost and snow for those sausages and other preserved delicacies. I could not understand it, why couldn't I enjoy them too, just as everyone else? It wasn't only that my responses were implying "don't eat it," when I did I later regretted it, even though I enjoyed the moment of eating it. I mean, I was not much of a vegetarian then so they tasted great, especially the bratwurst, which came hot grilled in a fresh baked bread roll with plenty of sweet mustard. How sad could I have been? So I ate the odd one anyway, just to test the effect, normally ending in my desiring to lie down and sleep.

Eating out in Germany was potentially good, they actually noted the food additives on the menu, but for reasons no one can explain to me they appeared obsessed with adding in to many things a food flavour enhancer called Maggie which it appeared at the time to be heaped with MSG, monosodium glutamate. Although I may be wrong on this, as I am now under the impression the product maybe also comes without MSG. That MSG stuff makes me thirsty for hours when added to the food I eat, and makes me drink a lot more beer than I might have (I'm sure the motive for adding it is not to sell more beer though). In

Shaun M Sutton

some German restaurants I have a feeling it gets added to a lot of things to add flavour, nice but unfortunately it's not for me. I would test salads, because of the potential for flavour additives in the dressing, by trying to hold my salad bowl and discretely breath test whilst sitting at the table, but my wife would nudge or lightly kick me under the table and say I was acting weird and I was risking being embarrassing for us in public, especially when this was whilst out having lunch with her parents.

Meal times out felt like I was playing Russian roulette, with all the preservatives, and artificial flavourings to hit me, let alone anything else wrong with the food for me. Sometimes I was lucky, and other times it blew my mind and I'd be near falling asleep at the table. Another reason for a kick or a nudge, this time for being rude and embarrassing, especially in consideration that everyone present was trying to speak in English for my benefit instead of their native tongue, and I was fighting with myself to keep my eyes open, just about.

During our Germany visits my obsession with testing things was maybe more of a form of mania it seems, in that some degree of panic would occur should I be in a situation where I was forced to compromise myself based on what my responses were informing me of. I considered the correct term to describe my general behaviour would be a neurosis, although a medical professional may have a variety of names with which to describe my condition.

We stayed a few nights at another friend's apartment, an old style ground floor flat in Frankfurt, whilst he was away. I couldn't sleep well in the bed. The next morning I took a nose about outside the back of the house and found there was a storage area for bicycles, all hanging from the ceiling, situated directly under the location of the bed. Could it be the metal of all those bicycles was to blame for my disrupted sleep? I had felt it something difficult to test for. Equally my difficulty sleeping could have been aggravated by our old former toxic bedding which we had taken with us all the way to Frankfurt, back in the days before our bed went all natural and response friendly, or maybe the issue was compounded by the combination of the bicycles and our former toxic bedding, as I see it now.

In this same apartment I was aware of being very concerned by all the metal in our friend's small old-fashioned kitchen. Metal was all around me where I sat at the table for reading and writing. That extent of metal so close to me definitely generated a degree of neurosis concerning it and anxiety over its possible effect on me. Radiator by the table, cooker, washing machine and dryer, metal cabinet doors, all in close proximity to where I had to sit. My senses told me that I could observe the negative influence of a substantial metal item up to about 5 feet (1.5m) from me, the closer the more negative the influence. Here I was surrounded at close quarters, pinned into the corner beside the radiator, but the kitchen was the only really warm place in the apartment to sit.

In this kitchen I tested old fashioned glasses with the bubbles in them and earthen ware crockery against more recently made and thought I perceived that the older allowed me to earth through them whereas the more modern had a lesser earthing benefit. I loved the old-fashioned decorative quarry tiled floor and felt it allowed me to earth well. Something else I tested was whether the more modern factory produced ceramic and stone tiles did not allow me to earth as well through them when compared with older tiles or natural stone and terracotta. But there is only so much a mind can take on board, and I was pushing mine, and the extent of my metals paranoia was affecting my responses so much at this time it is difficult to differentiate what was real from imaginary.

I wrote my reflections, in a journal of this time at the kitchen table next to the radiator, as being amongst the most challenging to me so far, in terms of concern about my responses to the environment. Equally it was a stimulating phase in searching for answers and seeking a way beyond the current man made environment to which my responses were seemingly at constant odds with, from electronic devises, metals and floor surfaces that did not allow me to earth. This was at the time of me trying to live by my theories of earthing and metals.

I could take charge of my trousers, but the rest of my environment was much harder to control in the way I wished for, especially in situations where I had no ability to influence that particular environment, and I just had to live with it, accepting my fate as a result. I desperately desired to find a home environment that made me more at ease with my surroundings, one where my responses would not be potentially in a permanent state of compromise, as back then it commonly seemed to be the case, like I was almost under attack from my environment.

We travelled to and from Germany by car, the route beginning in Calais, France, then through Belgium and finally down half of Germany. It was in reality a fairly short journey of just over 6 hours to Frankfurt, but was quite hard on my responses and general condition. I slept often, exhausted by the car and road, and early morning starts. My breathing and pulses when checked during this trek were unbelievably compromised, the pulses were hard like a stone and the LAPD was commonly down to 4 or 5 whilst on the road travelling along the Autoroutes. I could hardly inhale with the diaphragm.

An architect designer friend of mine in Frankfurt once asked me what I thought of tarmac, or ashphalt, road surfaces from my testing view, when I was first explaining to him my early observations upon our material world. Good point I thought, and on testing ashalt in my leather soled boots, the black stuff proved to not allow any earthing at all, just like on a plastic surface. However only ashphalt is used in far greater expanses, on the roads, and parking areas, not forgetting children's play areas. Second to a certain commonly used home fabric and fillings material, I think ashphalt has to be close to the top of the list as the next greatest hazard to my own responses with potential for a societal issue. Concrete I found was in fact a good earthing surface from the response perspective. Everything has a place but we can have too much of such a useful thing.

During the drive through Europe to Frankfurt one can find the odd sections of concrete road, which I felt I benefited somewhat from driving upon, even though, according to my own theory, the car tyres are insulating it and me from being earthed. On these concrete sections I felt far less sleepy and tired as compared with driving on all the ashphalt sections. In Germany there were a few sections of Autobahn which had a concrete trucker lane, so I would often drive in this whenever the chance presented, even slow down in them and be happy to feel a bit restored by the experience, then race like a crazy man again when it was back to the ashphalt stretches to try and get the drive over with as fast as possible. Fortunately this is possible in Germany with more liberal speeding limits often being available on stretches of the Autobahn.

The more lanes of the Autobahn the more exhausting, and the poorer my pulse and breath responses when checked. The better sections were in fact when driving through Belgium, where there were a lot more big trees growing at the road sides to hang over the hard shoulder emergency stopping lane, as well as trees growing in the central reservation between the two directions of traffic. Having trees close noticeably improved my breath and pulse responses as compared to no trees, but when it came to those wide ashphalt stretches with the hard shoulder added to this, these were the nightmare sections. In Germany the drive was made worse, as efficient road management system chopped down and removed most of the trees from close by the Autobahn, at least along the sections we drove.

During the drive I was generally delirious with exhaustion, and commonly incapable of driving safely, so my poor wife did most of the driving, especially on the German sections.

Through my wife's prior design connections we were able to gain access to the reference library of the 'Rat für Formgebung,' the German Design Council, at the Exhibitions area of Frankfurt. This for me was a big step, delving into the greater and more significant world of designers, those individuals imagining and creating the material world I was being challenged by. I felt honoured to be fortunate enough to have such an opportunity, step inside the beast I was battling with, and happy to have the support of my wife in the little fantasy world I was creating.

We explained to the kind and helpful Frau in charge of the reference library that we were conducting some research into natural and sustainable design, materials and products, for want of a more appropriate subject title. Our Frau gave us a slight sigh of disappointment about our requested subject, like it was something tedious. She then told us, in German, that the previous year had been the year for 'Green and Sustainable Design'. I think I managed to get the gist of what she said about sustainable and green design. In her world of professional and world class design, green and sustainable were commonly the labels attached to lame or weak design, design of dubious quality, making more of what they were by way of adding 'Green' to the credentials, like a marketing gimmick. It possibly appeared so to the professional design world, many substandard products and designs where being laundered under this 'Sustainable' banner, to an extent of being a mockery within the profession. The Frau may need to correct me on my take on what she was insinuating, but it all sounded fair and reasonable enough comments to me. Upon inspecting the Green and Sustainable Product Design catalogues she provided us with, I think what I ascertained had been correct. Green and Sustainable Design was arguably being labelled as 'Please do not take this seriously, it's just a sustainable gesture I'm making to the world with this design, and by you if you buy into this', by way of its own presentation.

I guess this was a situation where some of the designers concerned had not really perhaps grasped the point of what green and sustainable should be about, such as being useful, and fulfilling a wider range of benefits perhaps. It was not clear if sustainable and green was being marketed to the more serious minded altruistic consumer, or just as some trendy waste of time fashion accessory. Or was it just that I was missing the point the information was presenting to me, being the range of possibilities offered by green and sustainable design. Most were impressively kind of useless looking, although I am not in any position to make serious comment on such matters really and I can afford to buy very little myself. At least this was sustainable and green rubbish, as opposed to planet unfriendly rubbish, which we already have so much of. I guess I was disappointed and hoping for something more inspiring, that's all.

We were able to spend the morning at the library, looking over books selected for us on products, materials and the processes involved in making more sustainable design consideration. We scanned everything and anything our Frau dug out for us, looking for something of interest in my own subject of how design affects us, and Design's response to this. Unfortunately what I was looking for was either too complexly described to be understandable for me, or I missed what I was seeking here. I also was a bit anxious at this stage over speaking of my real research intentions, for fear of the looney label being attached to me in this serious and prestigious design environment, and my wife becoming labelled by her professional peers as 'the partner of the looney,' plus there were the restrictions of language. Maybe if I had have been clearer in my request I would have been able to find something in line with what I was seeking, but I did not really know what I should ask for, without sounding vague and weird and a bit pathetic to be honest.

The most we were able to come away with were notes on a variety of models for managing and considering a sustainable design basis with environmental concern, which whilst fascinating stuff was a bit too intellectual for me to make sense from and was not what I was looking for, plus some interesting information on novel natural materials. I was seeking a confirmation that I was not actually just going crazy by taking notice of my responses, but unfortunately still found nothing to support arguments otherwise at the Design Council of Germany library. The search for something to confirm that there may be something in my testing of the world, by way of response in my breath and pulse, needed to continue.

Whilst in Frankfurt we were fortunate enough to get tickets for the prestigious German Design Council annual awards presentations. Very interesting to observe the world of Design and how it was functioning, but green and sustainable didn't particularly feature, this was mainstream stuff, yet nothing to suggest this current design world was going to revolutionise ours and shake humanity to the very core of our existence. These days did seem to have once existed though, and within German Design, associated with an era past within the strength of personality and charisma in earlier designers presenting world changing Design. One such designer I found reference to was Dieter Rams, formerly of the Braun Company.

The London Design Museum and the Goethe-Institute in Exhibition Road, London, together put on a joint panel discussion of Design Industry experts from both the UK and Germany to examine the impact and implications of the work of the designer Dieter Rams. Whilst going through this phase of Design investigation my wife had said Rams was the man all designers in Germany had learnt about, and so she had made the discovery of this talk. We went along for me to learn something new.

Rams had headed up the Braun Company's Design team for a period of time from the mid 1950's, leading them to win a number of major awards for a variety of household and kitchen time saving products, for which Braun became famous, revolutionising how people lead their lives. One major development of Braun's was the hand held hairdryer (I'm not sure who originally came up with the idea for this though), revolutionising hair dressing via Vidal Sassoon. He also developed his own modular shelving and furniture systems, something my wife always goes on at me about, that this is how design should be, flexible, re-useable, add-on-able, providing a basis for timeless design classics for the home that are accepted as art and something to be handed down to the next generation.

Rams made himself renowned in Design through issuing his manifesto for good design, his 'ten principles', and for such suggestions as "question everything thought to be obvious," which rang a few of my own bells, and "less and more", which presently feels like the opposite of what it is I am trying to work through here. The panel chairman asked the audience in their discussion to make suggestions for what could be the 11th Rams principle, to bring the principles for good design more up to date.

The Ten Ram principles were just what I was looking for in a way, just to help me understand how our world ended up how it is, at least for where my responses were concerned, and as a reflection of where society has been in terms of design

Shaun M Sutton

consideration. Rams's good design principles are that design should be:

- innovative
- makes a product useful
- aesthetic
- makes a product more understandable
- unobtrusive
- honest
- long lasting
- thorough down to the last detail
- environmentally friendly
- as little design as possible

When we got home after the panel discussion we chatted upon our interesting evening. I tried putting together my own statement for the 11th principle for good design as "improves the senses of the user". I might now say, "is friendly to the breath and pulse responses". I am not sure I would propose "is good for the health of the user", as health matters are a bit of a mine field for me. Therefore my own 11th principle for good design is currently

"is friendly for the senses and responses of the user".

However I can think of a number of cases where there is no user, so added to this could be, "where there is a user of the product design". It's perhaps a bit too complicated though. I'm thinking of all the situations where it could be difficult to achieve this without a dramatic change in how we live our lives, or maybe I am just barking up my own tree here? There are so many variables involved in the responses I am not sure how anyone could agree on how to design according to them. Then it hit me, and pulled me out of my tree. Again, what if nobody else is aware of their own responses? And let's face it, as far as I'm aware it may all be that it is just me and a mental disorder I am suffering from in the end. Other's may respond but remain simply unaware and maybe do this differently to me.

Without anything being clear on the value of making purchasing decisions according the senses and responses, and the limitations imposed upon these by our existing clothes, living and working environments and lifestyles, which are all seemingly not orientated around the needs of the senses and responses, getting designers, manufacturers, marketers and consumers to seriously consider these proposals is well, humm, possibly pretty well much of a non-starter.

My wife said she once heard a good lecture by a leading designer who said there were many great products designed yet they failed to be successful in the market, not because they were poor design but because people could not appreciate their value and application. This could be the case in this situation, great idea, but nobody can either get it or feel it, or see any benefit, which might not even be there to be seen. She also said that designers can be a little too caught up in their own professional standing and beliefs to be accepting of anything coming from outside the profession, from a non-professional in their own eyes, the likes of me specifically. Let's be honest, in Frankfurt I would probably get laughed all the way back to London, and from London, maybe all the way back to my village in the countryside where I grew up.

Just taking into account all the things a designer needs to take into consideration when designing a product, thinking of the Rams ten principles for instance, add this to the management and design issues for making design more sustainable, even though considering the environment is a part of the Rams manifesto for good design, then add in the needs of the senses and responses, this all becomes quite a long shopping list for the designer to take into their consideration and possibly makes the design process thoroughly more complex. Complexity equals cost, so the benefits need to be quite worthwhile and a visible reality. Yet the benefits of designing for the responses were not clear. This needed more thought.

Maybe if designers themselves changed their own trousers and started living more according to their own senses and responses, they might be able to see the potential in this. One German designer told me that he was fed up and not so stimulated by designing products that he considered as 'just churning out things that he personally saw no value in, but it paid the bills to keep the office running and a roof over his head, food on the table, the kids in clothes and supported in study sort of thing'. I am left with the thought that the interest is there within the chain of people involved in designing around such a concept, but my feeling is one needs to work on oneself first regarding the senses and responses to be able to work the broader issues out, that is of course if the responses are generally there to be observed by others.

Part VI

'The X-sensory response system'
Seeking a framework theory in support of observation

Whilst I now feel loathed to suggest a theory, this is more of an observation, and so it is open to being altered according to any further observations.

The 'X-system' is the abreviated name I've given to a plethora of sensory changes and body response observations occurring during the treatment process, from my view as an acupuncturist, which includes changes in the pulses and breath as well as encompassing all other simultaneously occurring reactions and responses in us, in line with changes in the pulses and breath. The system is of importance here because it allows me to tie in my own responses to the environment, including of course my trousers, into a bigger and broader picture of things. The full reference name here is the 'X-sensory response system'.

The thing is, I could not find the name for what I was working and observing, so this is the one I've made up, even though I am under the impression that there are a variety of scientists or other therapists out there speaking of something similar with different names attached, or using some fancy name which really doesn't fully grapple what this all is about, but I only say this because I have not actually heard of what it is commonly named. So in this situation I could also refer to this 'X-system' as 'Shaun's fantasy survival system of an elaborate imagination', in hope of getting the point across that it is a made up name and I am not a person of sufficient scientific merit to go around making up names for something of such potential significance.

For instance a therapist friend in Germany mentioned to me how what I was working with was in fact 'Bio-resonnance', which sounds like a fancy name for marketing this under as a therapy, but I don't know anything much about what that therapy entails, and it may go under a different name in the English language. But the point is there will be many names out there for this, all referring to the same thing, or to different aspects of the same thing.

Personally, and of course, I like the 'X-system' in abbreviation, as a reference name appropriate by way of the system being something vague and hard to fathom or fully comprehend, at least for me, X as the unknown. X as a symbol also denotes a crossing over, or meeting, linking up from different directions, which this is also all about. Who knows the name may stick, but the name is unimportant, call it what you like, as there must already be plenty of other names out there for it I am certain, as well instruments by which it can be measured.

I may have been somehow inspired towards using this particular name by the work of an eminent Japanese doctor and notable acupuncturist, Dr Manaka Yoshio, (1911-1989). After originally practising Western medicine, Dr Manaka became interested in oriental medicine, and in particular acupuncture and the meridian system for the treatment of his patients. I had studied much of Dr Manaka's acupuncture work, and was working with the theories he had taught in his book, 'Chasing the Dragon's Tail' published by Paradigm. So I think Doctor Manaka really first came up with this name for something of his own observations, which he referred to as the 'X-Box'. (Now days X-Box is the popular brand name for a computer gaming system, which is nothing to do with Dr Manaka)

Dr Manaka's X-Box referred to the way acupuncture meridians paired up to manage the whole body picture from the perspective of an acupuncture treatment. In my own therapeutic work I found that when treatment of the meridians was successful the breath became fuller, easier and more relaxed in applying the diaphragm, the pulses more even and calm, and the physical complaints of pain or restriction in movement would noticeably lessen. As noted earlier the observations of changes in the breath during treatment, as a consequence of treatment, appears to be a generally acknowledged phenomenon amongst a number of practitioners of oriental medicine.

In short where the 'X-sensory response system' is concerned, anything that impacts the upon the breath and the pulse is therefore also impacting upon the physical form of the body, through tensions in the musculature and associated with the meridian system, itself being just another reflection of this X-system. This is perhaps the basis of how acupuncture therapy may work on a physical level, at least in my own mind some aspect of it.

However the X-system is broader than just physical response, it is encompassing of all the responses occurring along with these of the physical, which indeed also provides a basis for how oriental medicine is traditionally considered as a treatment means for a wide variety of disorders of the body and mind.

The X-system is a two way system, in that we sense and then respond through it, and it is how we sense and respond in subconscious nature, and certainly beyond just those mechanisms generally recognised as being a part of the autonomic (parasympathetic and sympathetic) nervous system, as much as I was becoming aware. Living organisms gravitate towards that enhancing their ability to thrive, in theory, humans may be among the exceptions. Plant leaves grow toward light, the roots toward water and oxygen, animals migrate toward what they need. Darwin maybe would put this sort of thing down to being a fundamental matter in the evolution of species, those most apt at adaptation will thrive and colonise their environment.

I am therefore under the impression that what it is I am trying to describe and link to my trousers, is our inherited ancient means of doing the same as plants and other animals, leading to improved fitness, health, recovery from injury and functioning more effectively, providing better survival patterns and a basis for human evolutionary development. Those with it survived, those somewhere back in our own ancestral development perhaps.

If looking at this from the view of the acupuncture meridians, if the meridians are under less stress, which is what the acupuncture treatment is aiming to engage, then the body would be experiencing less physical tension and tightness. And again, along with this are the great many other things one could, according to traditional classics and texts, consider treatment of the meridians can affect from a health perspective. When the breath and pulse responses improve this reflects an overall improved functional condition, and an improved condition of the meridian system as one aspect or part of the X-sensory response system.

That's a very technical way to describe something so basic really. The X-system is how we change as a complete organism according to responses to our environment, and in man's past history when the human was evolving towards what we are a very long time ago, this would have been how we best found the path to enhanced opportunities for survival and subsequent species protection and procreation.

My observations of the leaves on trees through my window, and counting leaves with more clarity in my sight associated with improvements observed in my breath and pulses, may be demonstration of an improvement in my perceptions of the outside world linked in with the X-system, to be able to see or sense things that mattered more clearly, those things that mattered in daily survival. It is more about what is situated between the leaves that can also be seen more clearly.

To test this point I went out and obtained an opticians chart from my local optician and tried it out upon a few patients before and after treatment, yet for some reason we could not perceive any measurable immediate improvement of the eyesight as a consequence of treatment. This was maybe some other senses thing going on it appeared, my seemingly improved vision. At night in my bedroom, before we changed to the nice new futon, I would look at a picture in charcoal sketch on my wall in the evening light coming through the windows, trying to make out the form and all the sketch's details with my foot out of the bed touching the floor, and then again under the covers on the inflatable mattress. I am certain I could see more of the finer details of the sketch every time when the foot was touching the floor.

As man has to some greater or lesser extent possibly compromised the functioning of his X-system, through not recognising how to take notice of this, potentially being life's early warning subconscious protection and guidance system, and by unwittingly practicing what reduces our ability to function by way of it, we end up with the way the world has developed. Our brains and intellect have achieved marvels in designing a world in which we can live as we do, providing us with the necessary survival systems to make up for our lack of access to our own senses and responses, our X-system. Our guidance and protection provided via the fruits of our intellect instead of through the X-sensory response system.

Intellect and using our brains in the way we do is like a fall back survival system, evolving out of those times when it has not been possible to utilise the X-system, as another evolutionary strength and character in mankind, and possibly to other animals as well I imagine. This is like evolving a reserve fuel tank for when the main one is empty, for when we aren't allowed to function at our best and work with the senses and responses to a fuller engagement of the X-system. The problem comes now, that as a species we created a world that only runs off the reserve. Are we missing the potential for running off the main fuel tank in our lives if we are not utilising the senses and responses? The human world developed beyond the need of our senses and responses, we get on without needing them. But at what cost, or more the case, what opportunities are we missing out

Shaun M Sutton

upon as a consequence of not making more from our old and rather ancient X-system? Still in there, ticking away, primed and ready to be stirred back into life again when the situation is right.

So that is the X-sensory response system, and I continued to spend my time trying to fathom out it's deeper significance, if there was one to fathom, and whether this X-system is not merely that fantasy creation from my own imagination but a genuine feature.

There are many tests currently available to test aspects of this X-sensory response system that I have heard of or tried out. These are including the regularly used muscle strength tests of the Chiropractors of the USA and Kinesiology, neither of which I know sufficient about to comment on and then dowsing, of which I know even less. Basically any aspect of the X-system will provide a means to measure the whole thing, so there are all manner of existing ways, and potential new novel ways, by which our senses and responses can be observed in action.

Equally each testing means is a way of verifying each of the other means as holding substance and any meaning, which to me is a significant point from the view for any therapist. If one means shows response, then all the others should also. The other important point is that they are themselves an aspect of experience, as opposed to theory, so can all be used to also verify the validity of any decisions in matters arrived at by purely theoretical means, as well as in determining the efficacy of other testing means for the X-system.

For me this is the greatest value in making observation of the X-system, as over the years I've heard many theories in my studies that have been somewhat absent of a connection to practice. This is an issue for any novice trying to work these things out. Our world is driven by theory often too far separated from the sense experience the theory revolves about to be of much genuine practical benefit. Einstein discusses about this gap between theory and the sense experience, and warns about relying on science based on theory not directly connected to the sense experience, in his book 'the Einstein Reader', in speaking of 'Physics and Reality' (1936), under 'Stratification of the Scientific System'. He writes;

"The aim of science is, on the one hand, a comprehension, as complete as possible, of the connection between the sense experiences in their totality, and on the other hand, the accomplishment of this aim by the use of a minimum of primary concepts and relations. (We shall call "primary concepts" such concepts as are directly and intuitively connected with typical complexes of sense experiences)"

I'm not sure why I'm quoting Einstein here, especially as how so many others seem to, with whom I may not necessarily agree, but it just seemed to support my own feelings, even though he was using these discussions in the build up to explaining his theory of Relativity, which is way beyond my comprehension when I looked at it. But I liked his sentiments on what poor quality science was, and it helped me realise how a great deal of what I had been studying in alternative medicine over the years was based on poor science, by being way too separate from the sense experience to be of any real value to the more novice practitioner. What I had been studying was interesting and encouraging, and held truth in some ways, but only experience could tie it to theory in practise, and experience is what the novice unfortunately lacks. Using X-system tests is a means to directly connect with the sense experience, a place from which scientific theory can become generated in the primary instance. For me as a therapist, and student of ancient theory, this was the next step, to be able to potentially validate theory with these tests and make more sense of it, and develop my understanding of why this or that is theoretically the case, and to make sense of my own judgements, when later referenced back to what old or ancient books were saying upon a similar set of observations.

Jake Paul Fratkin OMD, of Boudler, Colorado, a practitioner for over 35 years, wrote, wrote of this subject from his apprenticeship with a Dr Moon of Newport Beach, California, in the North American Journal of Oriental Medicine, NAJOM, March 2012 issue. Jake spoke of Dr Moon as having learnt the muscle testing of Applied Kinesiology used by Chiropractors. Dr Moon, another Doctor of Oriental Medicine, used these muscle testing techniques to confirm a myriad of discoveries relating to oriental medicine, from the effects of different colours in front of the patient to see which made them weak, to proving the bad influences of: wrist watches, electro-magnetic fields and even negative patterns of thought. Jake said the list of things Dr Moon tested was endless.

In my own studies into the work of the Japanese acupuncturist Dr Manaka, we learnt of a Dr Yoshiaki Omura's 'O-ring test' that Dr Manaka used to confirm

Shaun M Sutton

the potential effect and location of treatment points for his acupuncture treatment. The O-ring test works on the similar principle of muscle strength testing, but just using the index finger and thumb of the patient made to form a circle. The patient pinches the tip of the index finger to the thumb tip with a comfortable pressure between the two. Then the patient would touch the selected acupuncture point with a finger of their spare hand and the practitioner tries to pull the thumb and index finger circle open. A good treatment point is one where the circle is relatively harder to pull open, whereas a poor point or location leads to less effort in excursion from the practitioner to open the circle.

A Japanese acupuncture colleague told me about another intriguing test which acupuncturists in Japan used to test things, simply know as the 'Finger test'. My friend demonstrated it to me, resting the pad of the index finger lightly on the thumb nail of the same hand and gently shaking the hand from side to side by allowing a rotation of the forearm back and fourth so that the hand waved a bit. The easier the index finger pad slides across the thumb's nail, the more positive the response to the test. I showed my wife the test, maybe I was shaking the hand incorrectly, I'm sure there is a more discrete way to do the finger test, but she indicated that I would be disowned by her if she saw me testing that way in public.

I read something about this Finger Test, and assume it is the same or similar as my friend had demonstrated, again in my NAJOM, issue July 2011, in an article by Peter Skrivanic , a D.Ac, of Ontario in Canada, and in the same issue another article by Cheryl Coull, B.A., L.Ac., a certified Shiatsu Therapist of British Columbia. Their Finger Test was developed by a Dr Tadashi Iriye from Osaka, Japan and then taught to their own teacher, a Ted (Tetsuro) Saito who the article said had founded Shiatsu in Canada. Again its use was considered for purposes similar as those of Applied Kinesiology and the O-ring test (also referred to as the Bi-digital O-ring test - BDORT) in the testing of acupuncture meridians and points, as well as the effectiveness of treatment.

Cheryl wrote that Saito made the 'finger test' on himself when he woke up in the morning, throughout the day, and last thing at night. He tested what he ate for breakfast. He used it to help diagnose his patients, students, family members, and even the family dog. He finger tested up close, and from a distance: the long subway journey to and from his Shiatsu Centre became his field trips. So were his visits to art galleries (he finger-tested paintings and sculptures), parks, pharmacies, and grocery stores.

There are more of these response testing methods that are used therapeutically, but I do not know that much of them. Many are used in the treatment rooms in response orientated therapies in order to learn of the condition of the body and the body's therapeutic needs to correct conditions patients bring, and for identifying when the body system (X-system) has been corrected. Others, like dowsing, I've heard of used for all sorts of things about the home. What I have been doing in using the pulse and breath is really nothing much different or new.

I have found it quite easy to make errors in my response testing, especially when the circumstances for testing are less than ideal, as I have mentioned. Having a variety of means with which to test the response of the body has helped me be more certain of the feedback I take from the tests. Again, where one test is positive, so too should be all the other tests. Some tests have advantage over others for certain situations and applications. What is being measured is something incredibly subtle going on in the body, so it is helpful to have a means of double checking the tests for this, confirming the effectiveness of both tests and therapies.

I guess this in some way described a lot of what oriental medicine has as its root, the root from which it developed out from, from the senses and responses, and was how the ancients came to know what they did. But many could possibly disagree with me on this as being too simplistic a view, and many more not understand what relevance this holds to our current ways and of western medicine.

At the time of me experimenting with my own forms of response test and in trying to pull a broader set of ideas together concerning medicine, it made me question what goes on to improve the body and the means and mechanisms potentially involved. Where my response tests were just measuring the subtler body response, could it be there are two therapeutic systems man is using therapeutically? One system on the level of the subtler response, of the whole body organism, via the X-system, and the other being what our Western pharmacological medicine works with, that of the chemical and other more direct physical means of influence upon the symptoms of a patient. Parallel yet unconnected systems managing our health. I asked a couple of more experienced practitioners a question on this: 'Could there in reality be two separate but parallel systems going on in managing health, the ancient subtle response one, and then that of the pharmacological, where the pharmacological benefits, for instance through those things keeping patients alive in intensive care units, are not perceivable by way of our ancient system of the senses?'. But I drew a blank on obtaining any answer to my suggestion. Was this too deep and novel a thought perhaps, or just a question where no answer was possible or even warranted?

Could it be that as a result of our world being driven by the systems associated with us running off the back up fuel tank, the likes of our Western medicine and its more direct pharmacological approach evolved, beginning as man's back up system of therapy, to later developing to become the principal system we use in our current turn of the 20th to 21st century healthcare? The problem, as I see it, is that if these are truly parallel systems existing to which we respond to in health, then we cannot pitch one as being superior over the other. For instance me saying Eastern medicine is the superior as compared with Western medicine, or others saying visa versa. This is something as a therapist I had been trying to resolve for myself over some period of time, and especially since I had been focusing on these subtle level responses, this so named X-system for maintaining my health and that of my patients. Maybe the idea of parallel systems helps me make more sense of how the world of healthcare operates.

In just reviewing all these arguments I think the best argument point to consider exists when a situation arises where one of these twin parallel systems support- ing us is being run in conflict with the other, then that creates a problem. That's what we have in many situations now, providing a basis for dilemma and politics associated within our healthcare systems, and that's way more complex than my poor little brain can sift through. That I guess is man's human challenge of future evolution, to make the best from each of the parallel systems without weakening either in supporting us. I'm sure it is even deeper than this, but I'm not clear on which ways.

On a practical level, as a therapist making consideration of the significance of this X-system, my hands on work with patients became more fully tied in with accessing the X-sensory response system of the body, by way of observing these changes, especially the responses in the body's physical form.

As for me when treating myself, using the breath and pulses had become my main guide at this time and a window to what was going on inside of me. How I was and in how I was able to treat myself in all my therapies, from working on meridian points, locating them and getting a sense of when the treatment had been successfully completed, to finding herbs that would exert beneficial change on my system, and in identifying when I'd taken the correct dosage to be most effective, as demonstrated by a dramatic overall shift in my X-sensory response system at that moment, with a multi-level set of simultaneously occurring responses.

I coin the concept of Mizutani Junji, a practitioner of oriental medicine in Vancouver and co-founder of the NAJOM, which I found helpful within an article of his. Mr Mizutani describes treating acupuncture points by 'spooning' on the dose of the treatment to that point until it is full or completed. I was noticing this phenomenon when treating myself, and could observe this via changes in the breath and pulse. When acu-treatment points were first located, by means of response testing, the moment that I had 'spooned' sufficient dose was when the pulse and breath would no longer improve when again testing the responses when once again touching that particular acupuncture point. This also applied for when I had been testing an herb or herbal formula, but in that case when I had spooned in a certain quantity, the most effective dose for that particular remedy, then the pulses and breath became as they were when I had merely tested that remedy. Changes in the X-system act as indicator to gauging when this most effective dosage has been 'spooned on', the moment when no further response is observed if re-testing with that same herb or formula, or acupuncture point. (For further information on the application of response testing in therapies refer to appendices 6, 7 and 8.)

Working in this way led to further insights of the X-system as a whole. Patients would commonly make comments at the end of treatment, and I would keeping hearing the same sort of words and phrases about how they then felt, at that moment, and began to experience these same things more clearly in myself whilst treating them, as well as when just for myself. These were those deep and meaningful moments, like the world and view on it had altered to a kinder one, as though nothing mattered so much any more, acceptance, clarity, all sorts of things happening with the brain and perceptions, as much as changes going on with the physical body.

All very nice, but where was this leading? It was some sort of vague open end so very far removed from the world of design and my toxicity issues to the materials world I was personally still living with. I began questioning the worth of my work as a therapist. Were we as therapists just spending our time trying to plaster over cracks in a wall of a house experiencing subsidence? I felt I needed to think ahead more, to identify and deal with the root of the crumbling brickwork, appreciate why the house subsiding in the first place? That felt like too big a deal to question, but could I ever consider changing profession, learn how to underpin the foundations and work outside of the visible problems rather than inside?

I drew an analogy to remind myself of this point. A boat is being sailed on the ocean and the sailor is forced to bail out water because the boat is falling apart, full of holes letting in a slow steady stream of water. The sailor is so busy in bailing out the water he hasn't time to work out where he needs to sail to or how to navigate the ocean.

This was my dilemma, I was seeing my own therapy work as mere working with a cup to remove the water, which whilst helpful in keeping the boat afloat, was I but a band aid if I consider the way people live and our living environment for starters. I was looking for a hole filling and repair therapy for the bigger problem, somewhere it must be out there, surely. I was tired of just being the cup man, I needed more tools to work with. Well, this is what I was thinking at the time.

Part VII

Experiences of Nature

Experimenting with grounding or 'earthing' myself for the benefit of my responses, via making a direct contact to the natural materials around me that were connected to earth, was without doubt some sort of obsession I had developed. Touching walls, wooden tables and skirting boards discretely, without attracting attention to myself, remained my regular practise. Of course my wife could mostly see it and allowed me to play in the way I chose with the occasional raising of eyes and shaking her head in disbelief over what her husband was up to in public places. It was a habit I practised all the time, which I had felt was especially necessary during our year of regular trips to Germany by car, this delirium inducing journey we undertook each month along the auto routes of Europe.

During our trans Europe trips we would have to make our stops and break, and whilst taking it in turns to stay with the car I was allowed an opportunity to stand about on the grass, or curb side if there was no grass, touching plants and trees whilst testing my inhalation count in attempt to gauge the sort of state I was in at that stage of the journey. I was always hopeful of reviving myself, even if just a little before going back on the road. On these occasions the thing I would notice was that after an extended time in the car my pulses would remain tight, hard and forceful, and wouldn't relax promptly even with my directly touching nature. I was tense and shattered on these long drives, which maybe explained the hardness of the pulses. I would take every opportunity I could in trying to bring my system back to life, and any direct contact with nature felt better for me.

On one occasion, travelling home through leafy Belgium just before Antwerp, there was a nice wooded area next to the parking places for a rest area we had made a stop at. My wife goes off to the ladies and I take the opportunity to stand on a patch of grass, enjoying the afternoon sun on my skin, whilst leaning against an oak tree, touching the tree's trunk behind me with my hands for a more direct to nature contact. Cars would drive slowly by me, the drivers staring a glance over my direction, which made me feel like I was being a little too obvious with my tree hugging, then park up and the driver take a walk into the woods just a bit further along (in all likelihood to save the price of using the toilet, a common practise at European auto route rest areas because of the 50 or so cents toiletting fee). I was always careful where I trod at these places, and never wandered too far from the car for just such reasons.

When my wife returned she said the place was somewhat odd and empty of people. It was strange to have so many cars parked here and yet no one inside the building. I mentioned in jest to her how all these guys were checking me out whilst I had been basking in the sun hugging my tree, and she suggested I did look like a bit of a weirdo hanging onto the tree in the way I was, and that should be a lesson for me to be less obvious in future. As we drove along and out from the rest area we caught sight of a distinctly odd phenomenon taking place in the woods, the place was full of men randomly milling about amidst the trees, experiencing nature. Our European brothers have seemingly already cottoned onto the benefits of stopping off for a recuperative break in the woods, whilst on those long and tiring journeys, and it appeared to us as a very popular practise, at least there.

This provides a good example of how easy it is for people to get the wrong impression of one's actual intentions whilst loitering about in natural environments. Staying in Frankfurt Germany is not the best place in the world to discover a full-on nature in the city experience, but surrounding this city are many broad stretches of wooded area. Trees were good I felt, having noted improvement in my responses when driving nearer to trees when they were present and closer to the roadside. One cold winters day we went for a long run through the local woods, bringing along with us my wife's parents dog for some exercise, a ginger Cocker Spaniel named Sven. Her parents didn't seem to take him out so much, other than for his regular toilet breaks.

The dog had a significant issue with taking instruction, just didn't or couldn't listen, running wildly through the undergrowth in his own world, unresponsive to our shouts and calls. After about an hour in the woods, with the dog running wild around us, I looked over and saw him performing his business (poop). Whilst we stopped and waited for him, I noticed the way the woods had previously looked visibly changing somehow. The tree trunks became more obvious in shape and shade, above a copper coloured carpet of leaves covering the forest floor. I had to look again to see if I had taken it fully in and allow my eyes to focus more clearly, the perspective of distances altering. The trees stood out more defined, they were more obvious, that was it.

Five minutes later the dog stopped again and repeated his business, poor thing. How could such a little dog hold in so much business all this time into the woods, no wonder he was so frantic, but from then on and for the rest of our run he was a changed creature, and not the same beast we had originally set out with. He was now aware of each instruction we gave him, transfixed on my wife, running along to her heal without a leash, no more running crazy through the woods.

A year later, this time sledging in the mountains after an unseasonal amount of snow had fallen where we were in the Black Forest of Germany, we were sledging up and down a long track, again in the woods with the dog in tow. About an hour after we had been in the woods I look round and the dog is making a major business, and once again all the trees are going weird in front of my eyes, standing out, almost leaping at me from the woodland, the scene becoming three dimensional from two dimensional, just all of a sudden.

I'm not certain of what all that is about, these were just several notable encounters made with the woods. It was not just how the appearance of the trees changed to me, but I recall an eerie quietness that came with it in thinking back to those two occasions. And then of course the dog, the cannot listen won't listen ginger Cocker and his bowel evacuations, and then afterwards becoming the most attentive dog you could imagine or dream for, instead of his regular deaf to instruction state.

A friend of my wife's, living not far from Stuttgart, had married this great guy Ekey, who worked as a nurse at the local intensive care unit and drove a Harley Davidson motorcycle in his spare time, his love second to his wife. They would look forward to our occasional visits from London, and always looked after us with the best and freshest fare they could source locally to celebrate our arrival for a couple of days. We were very fortunate of such reception. A couple of summers ago we again dropped in on these friends, in time for the celebration of my birthday in our usual fashion.

In chatting with Ekey over an outdoor breakfast in the sun, I asked him if he had yet finished the higher nursing studies he had been struggling towards over the past few years. He said he had, informing me that the studies had been towards a project on the care of the relatives of those looked after in the intensive care unit. Ekey said that his project's conclusion was that there needed to be a special area in the hospital set aside for the relatives, whilst they waited upon news about the condition of their loved ones. This was a subject I was indeed very interested, with all my toxic environment thoughts and theory, so I commented that such a room should be set in a nice natural environment, or maybe with a garden attached. He agreed but said whilst he had the same idea also, generally these sorts of things were kept on a tight budget and it would probably go ahead with a token gesture of attention along these lines. He then went off for a moment to return handing me gold, not quite in the literal sense but to me this was what I'd been seeking for months, maybe years, perhaps forever.

The gold was in the form of a book his brother, a professor in horticulture, had co-edited for the 'Proceedings of the Eighth International People-Plant Symposium' on 'Exploring Therapeutic Powers of Flowers, Greenery and Nature'. The book was made up of the presentations given at this genuine and seemingly quite prestigious event held in Awaji, Japan, in 2004. The book, published by the International Society for Horticultural Science, was Acta Horticulturae 790 of June 2008.

Shaun M Sutton

Subjects covered in the recording of these lectures, provided by a variety of international specialists, were on how plants benefit humans, from plants as medicine, to presentations upon the benefits of gardening, courses studying horticulture as therapy via distance learning, rehabilitation of the sick and recovery from trauma through being exposed to plants or participating in horticulture, etc, etc.

Ekey said I could have the book as a birthday present, but not to tell his brother should we ever speak because it had been a gift to him. I was simply overjoyed. Could the study of plants and nature, from a therapeutic view, possibly provide me the missing part of my the puzzle I was working upon, and become e key piece to knitting together a bigger picture I was seeking for my own observations and responses?

I was excited to learn something of a subject so potentially significant which I had never encountered before, although I did have a patient who was in fact working for a charity within London in this line of work, but I had not acknowledged that relevance until discovering 'Horticulture as a therapy' for myself. The surprising thing is that I had actually studied horticulture for four years at college, after my final school exams, but had left the profession after working in it for a few years because back then I'd considered it as being a bit too unsexy as a profession during my youth. Now to me horticulture appeared as the sexiest profession on the planet since reading all these fascinating presentations on the things to be gained from working with plants.

Within the mass of articles of the Awaji People Plant Symposium report was one about studying horticulture as a therapy via distant learning in New Zealand. For participation on this course reference was made to a recommended reading book titled, 'Green Nature Human Nature - The Meaning of Plants in Our Lives' by Charles A Lewis, of Morton Arboretum, 1996, published by the University of Illinois Press. This book was presented as being the book that began this movement of thought on 'the human response to nature'. So I ordered myself a second hand copy from the Internet.

Lewis's book provided many gems of information, including research showing how patients in hospital rooms with a nature view recovered more quickly than those without such a view. But the most important part of the book to me was Lewis's discussion upon the seminal research carried out by two Environmental Psychologists, Rachel and Stephen Kaplan of the University of Michigan, Anne

Arbour, presented in their own book 'the Experience of Nature - A Psychological Perspective', published by Cambridge University Press in 1989. I had not been aware such a profession as Environmental Psychology had existed, or even what it was about.

The Experience of Nature provided details of a long-term research project monitoring the experiences of participants on outward bounds trips into a forestry wilderness site over a 10 year period, and documenting these from a psychological perspective. The portrayal and discussion of this research made up a major part of the Kaplan's book. The outward bounds trips were each for 10-14 days, during which time participants built up survival skills in preparation for a solo experience in the woods, being on their own for a few days in the deep forest. Every participant was encouraged to maintain a personal journal for recording aspects of their experience whilst spending time in the woods. The Kaplans presented some of the key words and phrases used in these 'wilderness inspired' diaries within their work.

It caught my attention that the phraseology and language, used by a number of their wilderness inspired participants in the study, had held a certain close similarity to my own inner language and that used by some of my own patients at the completion of each treatment with oriental medicine. Finally, had I found a link to something else, beyond that of my own profession, sharing the language I was looking for, perhaps the language of nature?

My own profession is considered as an alternative form of medicine to society, meaning to treat disease. My feeling was this placed a limit on how people viewed it, limiting it to disease and symptoms, limited by our own awareness and reasons for receiving it, indeed even missing a much broader potential I was attempting to investigate. To find out nature perhaps had the same effect on the mind as my own work with oriental medicine appeared to achieve my ends, and provided a potential breakthrough to me.

The Kaplan's book was a bit too expensive to purchase second hand, however I managed to locate a copy at my local University library and copied key parts to study and make notes upon at home. I then discovered, through Stephen Kaplan's own web pages, that I could order the book new through the Michigan State University book sellers, Ulrich's, which I then contacted and procured my own wonderful copy.

This marked entry into my Environmental Psychology phase of research, visiting the local University library regularly to copy any articles I could find from the profession's journal, on anything remotely mentioning of the benefits of nature, or how design influenced human psychology. I purchased a few books on the subject, including Environmental Psychology for both Design and in the Work-place.

Yet, the research period ended with me still considering the Kaplans 'Experi-ence of Nature' to be clearly the best information I had come across for me, in spite of its age, in making the link to where I was at and the broader perspec-tive offered by nature. They had recorded all their research protocols, provided copy questionnaires to be completed by their outward bound participants in the appendices, and given a wonderful insight into their work, how they had put it together and their own thoughts upon its significance to humankind.

The work did not introduce into it anything about the senses and responses, which I was especially interested in finding associations to in another profes-sion and make further link of my own obsevations to something beyond oriental medicine, although they did introduce 'Attention Restorative Theory' to sum up discussion on how mental fatigue is countered by nature's restorative potential upon humans, and provided some link between their work to 'X-system' theory.

Following up further on this lead with Environmental Psychology, it turned out that the University of Surrey, virtually on my doorstep in Guildford, has one of the world's leading departments for the subject. On visiting the course web pages I noted that there was to be a special lecture presented by one of the depart-ment's Professors, a David Uzzell, as a joint British Academy/ British Psycho-logical Society venture, held at the Royal Society of Greater London, in Septem-ber 2010. So I obtained a ticket and went along, having just noticed the event a couple of weeks before it was to occur. The lecture was titled 'Psychology and Climate Change: Collective Solutions to a Global Problem'.

I was interested to learn something more of the current flair and presentation of Environmental Psychology, given my interest in the Kaplan's theories, to consider the continued potential for a link to my own work with senses and responses. I would like to excuse myself if I report the event differently to how it was intended in consideration that I am not an academic myself, and in full respect of that profession, on which I know little other than what I gleaned through my personal study during that time of investigation. I trust I reasonably got the gist of the lecture as this, which remained my reflection noted at that time.

'With the world becoming generally more concerned over some potentially detrimental environmental changes being reported upon, Environmental Psychology, by way of its name and special placing as a profession, had secured substantial research funds to investigate why consumers were not making purchasing choices for more sustainable and environmental reason. The talk was interesting and enlightening. The conclusion, which I hope I am correct on, was a little startling to me. There was suggestion that because of the genuine and real concerns over global warming and change issues, if consumers didn't start to choose the more environmental and sustainable options available, then Governments would eventually be forced to regulate such changes as mandatory'.

The mention of regulation unsettles me, with the risk of state and law acting to limit personal liberty and freedom is my impression of many such regulations. Perhaps that had been the intention of the Professor, to stir the audience, stir those present to think and act more considerately in purchasing decisions. Is it that regulation, the necessary evil to protect ourselves from ourselves, adds a great deal of unsustainable practise within the bureaucratic processes of managing and policing the regulatory policies? But I'm a bit of an anti-regulationist, for my own reasons, so I cannot deny the negative emotions this conclusion generated for me. I was stirred, anything but more regulation please.

I came across another book given to my sister in law, by my own sister no less, when I visited their home. The title attracted me, 'Listening to the Land', published by Chelsea Green and written by Derrick Jensen, detailing interviews made with leading Environmentalists considering their thoughts on sustainability, environmental projects, their theories, experiences on nature, culture and eros. (I'm still not sure what eros represents in this). The book interested me, so I borrowed it, and in fact I still have it.

'Listening to the Land' was captivating, but nothing much really clicked for me in it in line with my own work, as being any closer than that of the work of the Kaplans, with the exception of the authors discourse with Linda Hogan, a Chickasaw Indian poet and novelist. Her conversation used language that connected in ways more familiar to me, language was her interest, specifically in relationship with the Earth, and in the transformation of loss and pain to becoming more whole. She explained her ideas on how English, as a language, was somehow limited in it's means to communicate about the condition and state of nature, English being more of a language designed for economics than for emotion, and that it is not a language capable of touching the depths of our passion, and of our pain. The native North American Indian, as a traditional race, has been through much pain during man's fairly recent history, which is expressed within Hogan's writing work.

I purchased second hand several of Hogan's books, including a book on short stories, 'Dwellings - A spiritual history of the living world', 1995, published by W.W. Norton and Company, and a book of poems, 'The Book of Medicines', 1993, published by Coffee House Press. Both books inspired me in how I viewed language, and even prompted me to begin my own experiments with poetry, observing the simplicity of how sentences could form together through having read Linda Hogan's work and then having a go at it for myself.

Finding this possible connection between my own work and others, within Language when portrayed through a connection with Nature, was the key perhaps and thus my next line of investigation. Significant for me was how it seemed as though I could now connect to the broader picture I was seeking via Language, to disciplines and backgrounds far removed from my own of Oriental Medicine; within Psychology perhaps, certainly through the Kaplans, and possibly also the language style of the North American native peoples within Hogan's work.

Nature was the key, is the missing link, it pulled me through this phase, Language my connection. It is easy though to get lost in a world of words, when without an appreciation of the place from where they came. The language of the bigger picture I was searching to connect with, and the same language of nature experienced when the pulse and breath becomes optimal, or the psychology underlying mental fatigue and of the fatigue free mind state described by the Kaplans in the Experience of Nature, representative of the same human condition of being from which the words have emerged. The same language as Traditional peoples, living closer to the beat of the Earth, and surviving without what we now need to live. Parallel worlds, parallel existence, lost world, lost history, forgotten until we again can speak this language of nature. I don't know, I'm thinking this in English, maybe that makes me overly logical in expression to connect all these things to the language of nature.

In Linda Hogan's poetry her language comes at times from a dark world associated with the injustices issued upon her native Indian people's past, pitted with horror, and a place from which it is conceivably difficult to see peace, possibility or freedom, even any hope at times. Yet from elsewhere in her work she was there with the rocks of the wild places and the home of the native creatures and peoples of America, representing the language and world of all native peoples quite possibly, and in English, our language of economics.

Maybe this is what the native peoples, the wild peoples of the world, are having to contend with, as the parallel world of Western man encroaches to their very core of existence, like contending with a disease, associated with the differences between parallel mind sets. There are many reports and documentations of disease in the Americas when the Europeans arrived, it is what is recorded as having destroyed their civilisations, through smallpox especially, as much as from the control of the gun. Was this plague linked to differences in mind set? Maybe not, but disease is much more than just chemistry and microbes from my own perspective. But really, could this disease be some form of a reflection between the differences in mind set underlying the language each civilisation was using?

I'm stretching reality perhaps, I'm going full circle, attempting to rediscover the wild within ourselves in the early 21st Century, through a language probably more designed for development and managing the ways of our current economic world, coming from the world parallel to that of the wild. It feels like I'm headed for deep water, and feels like it's potentially quite easy to drown within a sea fed from the streams of my own sentences.

From the 'Einstein Reader', by Albert Einstein, 1941, on 'The Common Language of Science', he writes

"What is it that brings about such an intimate connection between language and thinking? Is there no thinking without the use of language, namely concepts and concept-combinations for which words need not necessarily come to mind? Has not every one of us struggled for words although the connection between 'things' was already clear?"

A man of science of old, perhaps able to speak in the languages of both parallel worlds, almost speaking the same language concepts as Linda Hogan, facing the same challenges to say what is wished to be said. Maybe Einstein was looking out of the window to countryside when he wrote this, as opposed to deep in some laboratory office tucked out of daylight's sight, my mind overcoming the stereo-typing of men of science developing their concepts from pokey corners without being able to connect to that other world, that of the wild.

Part VIII

The Language of Nature - Part I

Loosing myself in the language of nature

As a result of being inspired by the work of Stephen and Rachel Kaplan, and the poetry and general thoughts about communing with the natural world in Linda Hogan's writing, I leapt into the hard to define and spiritual for clues linking my working with the responses into a bigger picture, and even further on from any medical consideration.

Explaining a relevance between my trousers and matters spiritual is perhaps no easier than linking them with anything else, but to go there feels a bit more risky. A journey across ice, thin in places, needing to be completed as lightly and quickly as possible, or by way of carefully crawling along on all fours for the oc-casions I may need lie flat should the surface begin to crack, to help save myself being lost to the depths below. It was a journey I felt compelled to take, rightly or wrongly.

Through working with the senses and responses of breath and pulse I had felt this association, in connecting my work with religion and matters spiritual, to be worth a look on some quite basic level. There is no way to prove any link here, and I already feel there is no value going down this path, which could be open or closed to argument.

However by way of investigation I made some months earlier, I had borrowed my family's old King James Edition Bible kept by my brother, to research for rel-evance between my own observations working with the responses and the early chapters of Genesis, to the purpose of looking into the descriptions on creation, the Garden of Eden, God, Adam, Eve, the snake and eating of the forbidden fruit. I took the step and peered into the Christian religion, that which I had personally grown up with as a child, in search for any clear associations to my work, taking a re-look at these old stories on creation I had heard at Sunday's school. This was a trip down memory lane, but in the same way as when re-watching a movie, it is surprising how little one remembers of the previous viewing.

During this phase of researching into Christianity, I joined my local Quaker church for a few Sunday meetings, finding them to be an easy to get along with community, and having some interesting dialogue with it's members regarding their tradition of sitting in relative silence for an hour whilst they met. I was also fortunate to have a former neighbour who enjoyed studying the Bible and had expressed an interest in joining me to read over the early Genesis, so together we were able to go through it verse by verse from 'in the beginning' to the part where Adam and Eve are cast out from the Garden of Eden by God. This part of the Bible forms the basis of discussion concerning the consideration of a relationship between God, our trousers and the senses and responses.

Before and during our handful of study Genesis sessions together, I could not help being struck by the thought that within the code underlying these verses of Genesis, God could be in some ways connected to this X-system, like a part of it, but I tried my best to avoid being too caught up on the idea that there was a relationship. Considering the broader intimation of religion or Christianity, which I know very little of, I chose to stick with my original research aims of what I was trying to ascertain, namely what else links to the senses and responses. Basically, I admit to feeling quickly out too far and that ice is awfully thin out there, and I've no idea how deep the waters are below.

However, before returning to my own metaphysical shallows, what particularly struck me from reading the early Genesis verses was how the idea of nutritional recommendation, on what is good for us to eat and what is not, has been around for a long time, it is there within early Genesis. Mankind's need for advice beyond what can be sensed for oneself is no recent matter, it is possibly just the way of how things are and have been for some great time by this account. I cannot personally see that we in the West have been much taught or encouraged to think and act for ourselves with our senses and responses as guide. It's just not something that has obviously been traditionally promoted. At the same time, I cannot see of anything to indicate we shouldn't learn to use and apply our senses. Perhaps they could bring us closer in search of God's instruction, or perhaps God to us is something completely different in significance. I leap for the shore, and scramble back up the earthy bank.

My next plan was to investigate whether the language of pre and post treatment reflection from patients matched experiences of participants to the Kaplan's wilderness research in 'The Experience of Nature'. I drew up questionnaires to be completed by my patients, using some of the same questions as used in the Kaplans research, to see if I could compare any observations between their work and my own. I began making records of the words that came up for my patients at the conclusion of their treatment, supplying them with a list of key words and phrases to be circled or added to when we had finished working in a session, to log the language they were feeling.

I continued the research exercise into the nature of this language used by my patients for about a year or so, but cannot say anything really conclusive came from it, other than it was interesting for me to observe how each patient completed their written forms, and how commonly those in a less than ideal way scored their health or made comments more appropriate to someone of a much better health condition. It appeared to me that words can be hard to trust and make judgement upon. It seemed that people can be naturally adept in fooling themselves and others to consider they are in a better way than they may actually be, likely a useful human quality, but to make it clear I know little on this subject.

Ultimately the task I had begun of a comparative research, between the results of my working with the responses compared to those recorded by the Kaplans, was a bit beyond my resources to comprehend or discover something useful from. Also I think it may have been a bit difficult for my patients, linking some of my more unrelated questions to their own therapeutic needs and concerns which were generally quite different. However, out of it all did come the most commonly indicated words used by patients at the end of sense and response guided treatments, being; calm, peace, quiet and peaceful, which were by and far the most frequently used of the 60 or so words and phrases offered to select from, and indicated as applicable in up three quarters of all responses.

In all reality I felt I was getting a bit lost in my language connection and off the point in all this, although it was difficult to admit to myself as I had been somewhat compelled along this road, but it ended in seemingly leading nowhere in my attempt to connect my sense and response work to something broader without my feeling the idea was now swamping me. I also hurt my back and started feeling a bit out of sorts, abnormally hot at night, having difficulty in sleeping through without interruption, becoming tired easily and just too sensitive to those things aggravating all these. Central London just plain exhausted me. It was common when meeting certain friends or patients for me to be left feeling knocked out from our encounter, and there were certain foods to be avoided at all cost, as no-no to my system for fear of crashing physically and emotionally.

More often than not I found I could pick myself up again, exercising outdoors with my daily Qi gong practise, or treating my meridian points with acupuncture techniques or using herbs, their selection and application always guided by my senses and responses. I found it would help to test my foods before eating, but I seemed not to be able to test all things all of the time, it simply felt too time consuming and tedious to continuously do it, like what a lot of messing about to cook a meal. Occasionally I found nothing worked for me, as though my whole system had gone haywire and the best remedy then was to just sit quietly, go pick up and read a good novel for a half hour or until I had really got into it, and then the responses were calmer after.

When I could not sleep I would get up in the middle of the night and treat myself with my own therapies, having the bit of a read if I had become overly mentally agitated, then go back to bed and mostly would then successfully sleep on. I regularly visited another acupuncturist for treatments at this time, for around a year or so, the style of acupuncture treatment different to my own methods. I hoped this might contribute to my becoming more open to the benefit provided by different therapeutic approaches beyond my own, try out something new to me so as to prevent me getting too closed to anything but my own ideas, with any luck, which I had felt at some risk of. But whatever was going on for me personally could not easily be abated. I think my acupuncturist was a little concerned for me and about what was underlying my symptoms and state of being.

I was being cut loose and I had to keep pulling myself back to earth, using my own senses as guide in this. In the end I came to the conclusion that I needed some extra help, as my own endeavours were not sufficient to turn me completely around, something was missing. All I could do was manage a bad job at best and keep plonking myself back to where I felt better before loosing it again.

Shaun M Sutton

Then came Christmas. I had a very stressful time with my in-laws in Germany, our individual worlds colliding, our thinking and sense of being appearing so far apart from the other's. We all got on as though the world was coming to an end and it was a strain for any of us to be conciliatory, especially me, I just wished to escape from them. I kept experiencing a re-occurring herpes virus, which I had had on and off for a great many years, the herbs I had available to take were helping, but no sooner as I cleared one episode from my system then another would flare up.

In practising my own Horticulture as a therapy I strained my back and gave myself a mild hernia from lifting some heavy compost boxes in the garden early spring, contributing to my growing list of complaints. I was falling apart and sticking myself back together the best way I could, but it felt like I was slipping backwards. Is this how it goes, life, is this just a matter of age catching up and normal ageing processes at hand?

About a year earlier I had visited some Kampo (see note 1) Japanese herbal medicine practitioners at their teaching clinic based at the Kailash Centre in London, being interested in the approach. At that earlier time I found the herbal formulas they had prescribed me with to be agreeable with my own response tests, so I went back to see what else the class and teacher could recommend for me through the Kampo approach.

I'm not sure if this is common for therapists to admit and own up to, but I think I had gone and gotten myself into a bit of a pickle really. Perhaps I had been overly concerned about all this trousers and sense stuff, perhaps it was the difficult economy so many were facing, which especially affected private therapists like I, or was it London and living here that just did not agree with me, or that I had difficulty in finding the clearer direction I was looking for in my work and doing too much of this research, or was it a culmination of the poor habits of my youth and age simply catching me up? Perhaps all of these or none of them were the cause, and all being experienced was just some cosmic response to planetary alignment unfavourable to me. Whatever it was I had to sort it out, by some means or other.

And so I began what ended up as nine months of fairly intensive therapy with the Japanese Kampo, regularly visiting the teaching clinic and using the traditional

Chinese herbal medicine formulas prescribed, gaining access to a source of experience beyond my own resource for the extra help I was seeking.

Note

1 In the book 'Kampo - A clinical Guide to Theory and Practise', written by Otsuka Keisetsu and translated by Gretchen de Soriano & Nigel Dawes, published 2010 by Churchill Livingstone Elsevier Ltd, in the Appendix 3 Glossary of terms reference KD168, Japanese Kampo is described as "Japanese herbal medicine, rooted in clinical use of classic texts from China's Han dynasty (203BCE-220CE) and enriched by cultural and medical experience from Japan".

Part IX

How toxic are the family?
And accessing 'a power-of-self'

In any discussion about toxicity, responses and our environment, it is easy to overlook and ignore the impact upon us of other people. In this matter I'm not so much thinking along the lines of how the behaviour of others visibly or tangibly impacts our lives, but more about the invisible connections and whatever else is going on there to affect how we are. I've no idea or theory on how it all works, all I can do is observe the end results and watch the interconnections from a sense and responses view, in the knowledge there surely exist sensible reasons behind this, all now mostly forgotten yet maybe more relevant than we can imagine.

My first introductions to all this interconnection stuff was in my Reiki training of about 15 years back, in which the level 2 part (I never made this second part though) did introduce and incorporate distant healing work. There was also a book my Dad gave me around the same time, which he had plucked out of a rubbish skip, the dumpster at the back of a second hand Charity store, him thinking it looked like something Shaun might find interesting (This store was not selling but disposing their book donations). The book was written by a Paul Miller sometime in the 1970's, and titled something along the lines of 'The Science and

Future of Spiritual Healing'.

On noticing this unusual book from the dumpster was published in Shere, near Guildford and close to my home, I drove to the address one rainy day back then to discover the location to possibly the world's original distant healing centre, of the late Harry Edwards famous for his healing demonstrations in the 1950's and absent healing work from his centre and home, the Sanctuary at Burrows Lea just outside of Shere. On one of my frequent visits to Harry's Sanctuary I picked up another book, this time written by Harry Edwards himself, titled 'The medium-ship of Jack Webber', containing a number of very disturbing photographs of odd stuff coming from the mouths of people sitting together holding hands, dubiously referred to as ectoplasm, in scenes replicating those more akin to be something from an old Hammer House of horror films production. That was all a bit of an eye opener for me back then, and still is now come to think of it. I'm not sure if this ectoplasm holds any association with the matter of invisible connections between people, but it does represent the idea of this all possibly be-coming a little too far fetched for many people to take on board. I still occasion-ally drop in to visit Harry's old home when I'm passing by that way and want to have a relaxing afternoon and get close up to nature, for it is a very peaceful place set in the genuine heart some magnificent English countryside.

Then there was another book I ended up with by a Barbara Brennan on healing, left with me by a friend Fiona who had made some courses with Ms Brennen. She could not fit the book into her suitcase when she left England on returning back home to Florida. She never came back for her book, or the rest of her be-longings I kept in a box on her behalf. Maybe she followed some intuitive instinct and left the book for me, maybe she just plainly moved on with her life.

In Barbara Brennan's book, I don't know the title as it's in storage, were a num-ber of drawings of people with all these lines drawn in passing between them, in different situations of encounter, representing the effects of human to human subtle influence. Her book was interesting back then, but ended in storage with many other books I didn't use, such as the one with the ectoplasm photos. I have to admit I was not able to make any real use of these particular books back then, other than them contributing in generating a certain paranoia about myself in re-lation to other people and their affects on me when I thought about it all. I think that's why it is in some ways easier to blot all that weird stuff out, and is perhaps a good thing if one does not understand or know how to deal with it all, as had been for me. I had an expression for it then, which helped me out, "if you can't close the can of worms, don't try opening it in the first place". As I said before, all this stuff drove me a bit unsure at the time, verging upon concerned about the side effects of my own shadow, and leading me to go study herbal medicine for the reasons already described, seeking the sanctity of others with hopefully not too dissimilar a mindset. And yes, of course I had opened the can of worms before I was necessarily prepared for what came out from it, or is that Pandora's Box?

So I tried to put all the interconnections stuff behind me to become more pragmatic about what it was I studied and worked with some time ago. However, since my beginning to make more and more treatment decisions according to the senses and responses, and less just according to some theory or other, I began observing the impact on a physical level of these human-to-human interconnections. Maybe I should go dig out Ms Brennan's book again, it could make more sense to me now.

So whilst I know my long suffering of my antics wife could be unhappy with an aspect of the following tale, on familial interconnections, and I wish I could tell it differently, the next story does thoroughly demonstrate relevance in this. During these times of my having sleeping difficulties my wife would snore quite loudly at random times most nights. It was not because of the noise this made that caused me to wake, I think I was already partially awake, but the occurrence of my fitful sleeping and the wife's snoring seemed to have some sort of pattern about them. Sometimes it was unbelievably loud and I had to laugh, really it was funny, there was no way to sleep during it. I wanted to take the phone and use its sound recording application to make a recording of her, because she would never have believed it was really her. I had a snoring problem too, it was a problem when I slept on my back but I liked to fall asleep on my back, it was more relaxing, and I guess she found the same.

I began by giving her a friendly little shake to wake her, or rolling her over onto her side if she didn't wake up to turn over herself at my suggestion. One night, I remember shaking her back and fourth with a little more vigour each few minutes, whilst she continued to snore in the deepest of sleeps with me lying awake wondering if this is a moon or planetary thing going on keeping me awake here. She just got louder as I became more frustrated, me oddly amused at my predicament, rocking her from side to side as she roared away like a beast by my side, eventually shaking her like a rag doll as I pushed on her shoulder forward and back, without any response from her, just the continuing snoring. I sat up whilst she was still going for it, there had to be a better way around this than shaking her awake. She always insisted I wake her up, but if she was sleeping and I awake then I felt we couldn't both be awake. I would usually then just head along to another room, read, treat my meridians, or take some herbs or all of these on more desperate occasions. Then going back to the bedroom to find all would be peace once more, almost always, she had moved on during that part of her sleep.

One evening, out of despair with the snoring, when I was just too tired to be bothered getting up and treating myself or reading in the other room, I decided to try treating myself in the bed, in the dark so as not to disturb her, to see if it would somehow calm down my frustrations over the disruption from the all this noise. Shaking her had not worked, so time to try out something new for this situation. I had been experimenting with some response driven meridian harmonising techniques in the treatment room, by way of my taking the pulse response whilst actually performing the techniques as a means to monitor progression as I went along in my self-treatment. I had been using them on myself previously but had not yet tried them out when in the bed, in the twilight. I guess it could be likened to an elaborate form of meditation, where I am observing how it goes through the pulses. This could be perhaps likened to a form of meditation for the beginner.

After 20 or 40 minutes, I wasn't watching the time, and towards the end of my treatment routine I was working with on myself, having already gone through a phase of there being something like a battle passing, between my finding calm and quiet, with that of the violent snoring generated by my wife, which in the dark made everything virtually vibrate, eventually she began to quieten, then with a final kind of croak she fell silent. A miracle! is what I thought. This became a new night time game to entertain myself about during the wee hours when I was awake and my wife snoring by my side. I still cannot understand how snoring does not wake up the snorer.

This snoring treatment result pattern seemed to continue, and around 8 out of 10 times I stopped my wife snoring, or this is how it seemed, by way of me just treating myself in the dark of our bedroom. At that exact moment of my pulses becoming calm, quiet and even, and my inhalation easy, she would stop, going quiet, then sleep looking like a baby and me too soon after. When this was not possible to achieve, and I could not win the inner battle, I would get up to read or do a more intense treatment than my simple meridian and pulse guided meditation. This was all much more interesting than shaking someone awake, which seemed a little unsporting now, and so I continued my new nightly sport whenever it was there to play, the game of could I stop my wife snoring though treating myself.

Of course the interesting thing about this sport is that my wife had absolutely no idea what was going on, she was in la-la land, yet I could generally stop the snoring through just focusing on what was going on with me. Such a phenomenon raises all sorts of questions including the ethical situation in all this, for instance me messing with my wife's snoring without her consent. At night I would think of such garbage thoughts and wonder whether in the USA this could be viewed as grounds for divorce, the tampering with the other person's processes whilst they were sleeping.

"Had your wife consented to you treating yourself in the bed to stop her snoring?".
"No, your honour".
"Had she asked you to wake her up?".
"Yes, that is so your honour".

I so often wanted to record the snore stopping therapy with a recording devise, but it was a hard enough to calm myself with all the noise of the snoring to contend with, let alone to add in messing about recording the experience. I think that may have been my mind racing too much to have considered the idea, but I was often tempted by the thought of doing it.

The question this matter raises is who is affecting who here, or are we just affecting each other, and who started all this in the first place? Hey isn't this the classic substance underlying most relationship argument and fall-outs? Certainly there were times when it seemed as though my own anxieties started to generate when my wife began to quietly snore, then as the noise slowly became louder, it felt like I had control of the volume dial to turn the noise up which was easy, but it took a lot more time to turn it down, and I could only manage it through my bedside mediation or a more intense form of self-therapy.

Considering all the stuff going on with me at that time, I was left concluding it

Shaun M Sutton

was in fact me who was the most likely cause of my need for these sleep time capers in dealing with the disruptive noise produced by my dear wife. I decided I was affecting her more than she me, or was I just being too kind in excusing her here? Neither matters. I was able to stop my wife's unconscious unsettlement through attending to myself, this was my role to play in this. Somehow this carries the important message to anyone in an intimately close relationship.

However, in treating my wife directly when she wasn't asleep I found it to be quite often a challenging experience. Mostly the treatment was for her having some stiffness, feeling on edge, anxious or not too well. It really did appear that her own condition affected me, or hey was that my condition affecting her, and it need be considered how I was just indirectly unsettling myself through my effect on her? However, if she was in a bad way it did not always seem to correlate I was too, and visa versa. But when neither recognised we were in a bad way that could spell trouble and argument between us, or me feeling as though I was treating her in a mind fog when I was working on her, and everything was much harder for me to sense and work out from her treatment responses. Occasionally the treatment just failed, which was not easy for either of us to manage. It is possible that living with me at this time was enough to make anyone anxious and unwell.

What I began to recognise was how I could sense this foggy mind problem condition, feel the signs in myself, and so I found it much easier to then suggest she should have a good run in our local park first, then later I could treat her when she came back. It was amazing the effect this had on both our systems, and if I did actually then treat her after her run it became a more straight forward job where I did not feel so unsettled in myself to read the responses, and avoid a poor treatment outcome. Treating her either side of her going for a run was interesting in watching the dynamics of it all and to learn of her run experiences. Often the case was that she could not run but walked before being treated by me, yet had an easier run if I had been able to treat her first. As a consequence of her just getting outside in the local nature, for an hour or so, a good affect was generated for her, and of course indirectly upon me, and we both felt a lot clearer for it when we were back together.

There was stuff going on but it was all quite difficult to exactly pin down what it was. However the general idea ended up as, if she was not in a good state this could be purely down to me, and instead of treating her I should go treat myself.

I had been making some similar investigation of patients and their families. Although I am not sure on the extent children can affect their parents via this interconnectedness, and have not tested to see if it works that way around, it became a fascinating project to make observations of how a child's condition and behaviour is to some notable extent directly affected by the treatment condition of their parent.

In fact before this time I admit to being a bit wary or even scared of small children. They were too unpredictable for me, like horses or canines, but making my interconnectedness observations cured me of this. They were simply little, and expressions of their parents, they could not help it. There was also the testing I made on couples for the extent treating one measurably influenced the physical form and body of the other. At one stage I thought that one child may be more connected to one particular parent, which may still be the case, but also found that treating both parents had a greater potential impact on the child than from treating just one parent, although I may be mistaken on this. The inter-dynamics and potential for implications from it all are quite intriguing and a bit mind boggling for me to think about.

These 'parents affecting the child phenomenon' observations all began with stories of children with difficult night time habits suddenly changing these after I had treated a parent, such as them wanting to sleep in the parents bed each night, or being devilishly behaved. Then when a parent was treated, as ever guided by the senses and responses, this habit would stop immediately after the treatment. In one case example after my having treated both parents they then phoned me from the car to say that on calling home to see how their home bound sick child was doing, with a nasty cough and fever, the granny said she had just a few minutes before suddenly stopped coughing and fallen into a peaceful asleep. This being at around the same time I had finished treating the parents, but about 6 miles away. Coincidence maybe, or not? It wouldn't be too hard to test the distance interconnectedness theory in practise.

I physically tested young kids and older children before and again after treating one or both parents. I would test one partner before and after treating the other. I once tried these before and after tests between two Swedish sisters but did not notice so much, just a slight something in one occurring from having treated the other, not as obvious as between partners or the parent to child response relationships, where a measurable change in the untreated parties physical tensions

Shaun M Sutton

appeared as significantly observable, and demonstrable. Time after time I continued to see the physical and visible changes going on in the untreated family members when there was an opportunity for kids to come along with a parent, or couples in a relationship to come along with each other.

Of course this does on some level make sense to us but we have not been educated to easily comprehend these matters as so, why should we, as we do not understand the mechanisms going on here. I'm guessing these interconnections, associated with what I think of as being 'a power-of-self', are a part of some ancient human survival mechanism, making families or communities stronger, fitter or healthier, more able to enhance their lives and then expand up their communities. I guess these matters are generally listed under ESP. Familial interconnectedness doesn't just have to be the negative observation, as recognisable in the inverse of the experience, but it can as such help explain away a lot of the difficulties families and couples go through. The interconnection dynamics, and repercussions within the relationships of others, are a real fascination if one really thinks about it. But it's going to be a bit deep and murky if it's about ourselves and how we are.

It is the child that misbehaves, blame them, cuss them, or it's my partner's fault, or the other's error. Of course it is, or not? How often do people look to themselves when observing problems in others they are closely connected with? We are not easily aware of these interconnections until the pulse, breath and mind becomes settled in us. Then and only then, do the interconnections really become more apparent to facilitate observation.

How far accessing this 'power-of-self', for want of a better expression, has potential to resolve issues in others I do not know and can only consider it as a possibility. However it is possible to do is as I have, finding some means or other to observe how others, intimate with ourselves, are influenced by our own condition, as much as how we, ourselves, are influenced by the condition of othes, when considering the senses and responses. Sometimes it feels unclear who is influencing who, but the best place to start has to be by working upon ourselves first and see where this leads us.

Part X

The Language of Nature Part II

Finding myself in the language of nature

"Hence it is said, 'the ancients who had the nourishment of the world wished for nothing and the world had enough; they did nothing and all things were transformed; their stillness was abysmal (deep and unfathomable?), and the people were all composed! The record says, 'When the one (Tao) pervades it, all business is completed. When the mind gets to be free from all aim, even the spirits submit"

From 'The Texts of Taoism - Part I', translated by James Legge, Dover Publications, 1962, as an unaltered reprint of the work first published by Oxford University Press in 1891, page 308-9 on The Writings of Kwang-tze (Chuang Tzu), originating circa 320 B.C..

Language in itself, what we think or feel, what others write or say occupies the processes of our minds and in one way is helpful, and yet in others is unhelpful. This started to become my conclusion in all this theorising as a result of my observations and reading the works of others, with a notion it all could assist me in finding where I was trying to reach, this place of pulling these matters together.

What was clearer and clearer is that there was no together at the end, in fact there was nothing, a big open nothing. I could theorise, observe, study all I liked but when it came down to it, my conclusion ended before even complete, and nothing was able to convey the final full stop.

This became the contradiction of it all, in seeking something I find it is not there, yet something is, just not what I had been expecting, nor even walking towards. It's not like falling off the end of a cliff, it's more like waking up in Egyptian cotton sheets after a long and arduous journey, smelling the fresh washed fragrance with the sound of the trees outside and seeing the way the curtains allow the light to dance at the open window.

I started letting go of even more things in my life, most especially my theories.

Shaun M Sutton

With each re-writing of something to describe myself, for the promotional purpose of my therapeutic work, I could not in the final analysis accept it, too wordy, too much bla-bla. Words were becoming unhelpful in containing the essence of what I did, was doing, and attempting to do in the treatment room. But words did help me out in a way. I discovered that I began to know the place I needed to find was that where words no longer exist, like sentences would just evaporate in front of my eyes to reveal a wordless world behind a veil woven in syllables. It was like running along holding a child, protecting it and then as if in a dream, as you continued to run there was no child anymore, you had no knowledge of where it went, yet you were awake and not dreaming either before or after the child had vanished from your grasp.

My primary focus developed to become be mindful of thoughts, ideas and even anything I wrote or exchanged in the world as being potentially out of line with what needed to be said, conveyed or acted upon. This was unless I was in a condition where my senses and responses were in their most ideal state, or at the least something close to as ideal a condition is within reason. I say this because I found I could waste a great deal of time on the unnecessary act if I was not careful when my condition was not ideal.

To maintain my condition I practised my Qi gong at least once a day, twice when necessary, and took the Kampo herbs prescribed at my consultations, as long as my responses agreed with the prescriptions. To my continual surprise was how I conferred agreement with the appropriateness of my prescriptions when double checked against my responses. As a therapist it was an enlightening period of sorts, discovering how my senses and responses agreed with the theoretically selected herbal prescriptions. I developed a lot of respect for the Kampo class for continually working me out correctly, or at least I was agreeing with them. I'm not too sure what they really thought of me, I'm a bit embarrassed to even ask as I was quite candid in admitting I would test their prescriptions before taking them, which was not normal and could quite easily have been viewed as being a bit insulting to their work, like I didn't believe them. Fortunately the teacher had confirmed having heard of similar testing means from colleagues in California, so I didn't feel so bad owning up to my checking the efficacy of their work against my breath and pulse responses. Looking back, treatment to correct me still seemed like a long old process though, with many phases for me to work through even so, whilst being pulled back from the brink of where ever I had been.

I would go out and completely loose myself most days in the nature spots within a cycling distance from home, loosing myself to the point of just sitting there watching the clouds roll by and thinking, hey I've been here before, with a welling up of a past distant location becoming significant. I would write poetry of a form, trying to capture what it was I had found in that place where my mind had totally disengaged. In some ways it was like catching a butterfly and putting it into a jar. You get home and it doesn't look the same, it's lost some of it's magic, connection lost to that place where you found it, now it's a little sad when you show it to your family, better it was free and not displaced from the world from which it came.

In this way I had frequent periods of time where I detached myself from myself, becoming no different to the trees, grass, or flowers I stood or sat with. It was a quiet place I was finding, quiet from myself, one where I was able to escape, actually from myself, or my parallel self, maybe.

I noticed all the fine details in these places, each flower or blade of grass, like viewed under a magnifying glass where ever I looked. Absorbing patterns in the movement of the field as gusts of wind blew across. Time became endless as it no longer mattered, I would often be made to be late after an adventure into these little pockets of local wilderness. Yes, this was still around London, finding the hidden, and easily forgotten corners where nature was reclaiming or has always owned the land.

When I took my herbs, carefully tested against my responses, I began to find it again, this new inner world much more quickly than when outside, that of the parallel mind for want of a better term. Emptiness would wash over my mind in almost an instance, peace, calm, and stillness re-establish themselves. It was like having had a party and sending the guests off when its over but the house is spotless, all cleaned up, and you are left with yourself, listening to sounds outside the windows and seeing a fine detail to shapes in the space around. When in the world of the home space it became a detached location for me when taking my herbs, like how did I get here? And then I'd wander off and get on with whatever I needed. Outside in nature the end point came with feeling simply a part of the place, another part of the scenery, almost as though I was no longer there, no longer human, unsure of from where had I arrived, as though I had previously been in some other world.

In the nature, following my senses and responses to direct my actions, I would end up feeling like I was a cat, or rabbit, or a fox, or something else that can just sit there, in quiet appreciation and contemplation of the sights, smells and sounds, responsive to each, no mind for distraction from his of her environment, living by instinct. Other days it ended with me feeling as though I was just another tree or a shrub, to the extent that I was feeling the language of the trees. I will admit to finding places so quiet at times during these nature experiences that if such a thing as garden spirits were to exist, you know fairies, if they had have been there I felt sure of being on the verge of seeing them at times, but in their language, this nature language. It was journeying to a new territory, to the essence of the natural world. To get there I had to forget, forget language, language could no longer exist for me. In its place was the world of the senses, and these visits were ending as an excursion of the senses.

I had read Aldous Huxley's "The Doors of Perception", my friend Malcom had recommended it. Each day I would have a new experience somewhat akin to Huxley's, without the assistance of mescaline as had opened his perceptions, or any other drug, just diligently following the senses and responses in what I was doing out there during these seemingly wild encounters around London. Then I would try to describe it in poetry, it was a place from where poetry came, a poetry fountain or spring. At this place a genuine writer or poet, or other artist would be able to capture a clearer picture, but for me it just allowed word to come with as little thought as possible. I was just interested to try to describe this alien place to my regular world the best I could. It was the parallel place, an uncommon world.

I felt compelled to do things and tried, but found that the most important were to consider myself as the priority before anything else. I became more and more self-focused, which I'm not sure is the same as being self-absorbed. I often noted the errors in my judgement when I was not completely self-considerate, wasting time then, time that could be better spent on just looking after myself I guess.

Sleep improved, no longer hot at night, less concerned over my trousers or their contents funnily enough. Sometimes I would find something in a pocket and realise that it had not harmed me in some way and that I had been feeling quite well. I'm not sure if it was that the sensitivities to the environment and foods that disagreed with my senses and responses had lessened, but I was getting better at keeping things in perspective. I was getting more used to the new territory of living in the knowledge of the senses and responses it seemed, there was a sort of double edged benefit thing going on. I was more accepting of the world, at least more than I had been.

My hernia resolved, I could handle central London better, even enjoyed my trips there. I would experiment with drinking the occasional real full caffeine coffee, a single shot Americano, but had to begin by taking care not to drink the whole shot. Attempting to settle my mind with Qi gong or meditation after a full shot of coffee could be quite exhausting and tough a job.

On the whole I began behaving more like a regular person, though still with quite a few idiosyncrasies in tow. I continued in testing things when I felt there a reason, and not to use anything my breath and pulse adversely responded with, but I got on more without so much concern or testing of everything I came into contact with.

In a way dumping off all my theories was a necessary thing, to define and allow myself to just evolve a bit more, they were from the time before and I was now a different person. My own self-generated theories and ideas had their flaws, which was becoming more and more apparent. So I began working more according to the accepted norm in certain ways, and being less of a maverick. I even began practising acupuncture with needles, as the potential benefit and interest of work-ing with them out weighed my previous metals anxiety and phobia. I just could handle working with them again.

I still find living in the current world often is plain debilitating, but know I can sort myself out, within the jungle of my own senses and responses. I see a place for both worlds, these parallel worlds in my life, the wild and the regular. Now I just need to get on and engage in life somehow, and discover what next. I realise the head and sense based worlds both served their purposes, as much as they are both useful to me. That's going to be the next challenge, at least for me, not to focus too much on one at the denial of the other. I now kind of understand how they both can help me out, help me in making it to where I need to get.

I have no far reaching conclusions to provide from my trousers. However, I hope this is more a tale to encourage experience than following theory.

Shaun M Sutton

Sitting out at night in the Autumn air,
moistening of all things to my touch,
droplets form on the branches in the mist,
sounds of their intermittent fall.

Translucent leaves turning gold from green,
still hanging on before the storms,
appear like a mass of yellow flowers overhead,
lit up beneath street's lamps.

The ground around covered with a thick scattering of leaves,
early fallen as winter nears and summer finds it's distance once again.
All is quiet.

Even the cars passing on the main road to town close by,
run seemingly silent at this time of night,
muffled in damp's lingering seasonal coat.

Thames geese and ducks go about their nightly business,
patrol the waters edge.
Night is their time,
they run this show from here on in,

And the river runs endlessly on.

Dilemma to change

Reflections arising from a bench by the Thames.

In Rachel and Stephen Kaplan's book that so inspired me, 'The Experience of Nature - A Psychological Perspective' of 1989, they added a final chapter entitled 'The Monster at the end of the book', in which to sum up their thoughts. Their work had helped me in forging my own connection between working with the senses and responses and a world greater, broader than the one confined to matters of medicine. It appeared as though through psychology I had found my connection as being the world of nature and its benefit to man, not just the nature for recreation and the aesthetic views it provides, but something deeper, a connection to our ancient selves from which the roots of my own studies of oriental medicine had emerged.

In their final chapter the Kaplans considered the situation of a small industrial country somewhere far way. One of the major industries of this country had for years dumped its waste product on the ground. There was now evidence that this material was showing up in the ground water. Further, it is suspected of leading people who drink it to be more irritable (and quicker to violence), less effective (and more likely to attempt to escape problems through drugs rather than to try to deal with them), less able to exercise self-control, plan for the future, and make thoughtful decisions. The authors suggested further to the reader that these people were experiencing an increase in various health symptoms and an overall decline in their health. The Kaplans asked if the country should move quickly to deal with the situation, and whether prudence would dictate that action be taken even if definitive evidence were not yet available?

It was considered in the Experience of Nature that decision making, due to the damage arising from the presence of something, in this case the pollutant, is somewhat easier to take on board for decision makers, than when the damage is due to a similar occurrence from an absence of something, such as the natural environment and the theme of the Kaplans book.

In Trousers I'm tentatively taking a next step, considering our problems are as a result of both the absence of some things that help us, and the presence of other

Shaun M Sutton

things that cause decline in ourselves. To which whilst this is an obvious notion let us add that we can work this matter out for ourselves, by way of our own senses, without necessarily being informed of it, or needing a dictate from other information sources to initiate our decision to act. That maybe sounds great, but it's also suggested here as being potentially a more dynamic and harder to grasp concept, having to go forwards on one front, yet defend and hold our ground on another. In making decision for ourselves, without someone other than just ourselves informing us, it is very testing of our means of coming to our decisions, as we do not have the habit in society of using our senses.

"Who told you this?", "Me, I sensed it!" To go through this the individual would likely be ridiculed to some degree by those who cannot sense and find it more straightforward to continue in the current ways of coming to decision and of societal determination. Whilst working with the senses may already appear to be a more complex concept, the decision making process could likely become confused further without a prior structure to include for such a possibility of including the senses and responses in decision making. We have to go forwards based on what is good, look back to isolate and exclude what is not desired, and manage our new way of making our decisions in a world unprepared for us, and us to that world. As the world has no structure for accepting such behaviour it could find it potentially irritating and difficult in all fairness to the world. Working with the senses and responses may in all likelihood uncover things challenging for the regular world to accept. Conflicts, aggravated along these lines, add to the burden upon the mind to find the quietened place in which to sense and read the responses defining how we view our new world.

The Kaplans have also made the comment,

"Confusion is debilitating and thus there exists the importance of maintaining one's orientation and being prevented from becoming lost". (see note 1 at the end)

Guiding oneself by way of ones own map to the world, uncovered through the senses and responses, is like feeling one's way around in the dark, at least that is certainly likely in the beginning. There are varying ways to consider this, including; as a result of being unable to see, one is then forced to develop the other senses to a greater capacity and extent of use. Or, alternatively could it be that by way of concerning oneself with and taking notice of what the senses are informing us of, would it be potentially unsettling for our organism, our system, our health even, through the confusion and disorientation this may generate? Or is this disorientation just a symptom of something else, like a mild hysteria, which can be easily calmed and quietened to refresh one's perspective, for instance through simply using the senses and responses further? Or does this kind of strategy simply risk one's sanity and health, lead one down a thorny path which maybe difficult to return from? In this instance it has to be asked, "why should one purposefully go loose oneself in the dark, why take your friends and family along for the ride, why risk one's sanity and health in all this?"

Becoming aware of our senses and responses takes up time, ties us up and is preventing of us getting on with our day to day personal and societal responsibilities, especially if taken too far, although I'm not sure of what too far means. As for my own motivations and actions, I feel I am saving time in applying the senses by way of making better decision through having engaged them, but don't know if I save more than I expend. Being accepting of any potential for benefit in this requires some degree of good faith in others who wish to give it a go or allow this for others close, which may be in short supply, and if it is considered as not being worth the trouble of upsetting and unsettling the status quo in an already uncertain world, too destabilising, its potentially viewed as too risky or costly to take a step toward this sort of change.

In the Experience of Nature the Kaplans introduced their own ideas on what potentially happens when we are deprived of nature, giving thought upon the mechanisms of 'fatigue directed attention' and mental fatigue, and what constitutes this in relationship to restorative environments and then again what it is that constitutes the restorative environment. This is now recognised as the Kaplan's 'attention restorative theory'.

In seeking the next step on, and through incorporating the mechanisms underlying mental fatigue within the broader view provided by the X-system, I hope to make sense of this picture being assembled in Trousers. Could it be considered that anything toxic could be detected by our own personal early warning systems before used, before we have lived with it, or popped it into our mouths, without having to have experienced its affects on us, experiences the like of mental fatigue for instance? Before having drunk the toxin containing ground water leading to the societal ills described by the Kaplans, could we hypothetically test this water contained in a glass with our own senses and responses, and would it have been possible to have spotted the pollution for ourselves? That is a key question

Shaun M Sutton

to ask, or do we need a certificate of purity on the bottle before drinking, and there again by what standards is that certificate provided? The problem is we take water for granted, I know I tend to, along with a great many other things including my trousers until fairly recently. But therein exists the problem, where do we draw the line on what we do and don't make a response test of, some things just have to be trusted, don't they?

Using the senses and responses may come across as a rather simplistic means to ensure one's health and good functioning in life, and as a quite basic means by which to detect what should and should not be trusted as appropriate for ourselves. Surely this is a rather naive notion to consider as there are many things harmful and compromising of our X-systems in today's environments, things we even need to take for granted in our lives, including our underpants and bedding for instance? If we had the time to test everything could it really drive us insane in the process, or would we be deemed insane by an unsuspecting world wishing to maintain the status quo, discouraging or preventing of the testing of these things in the first place? Should this be a good reason to not test things, just in case we go insane or upset others through our questioning, and loose our existing good status and standing in the process, or risk injury to our intimate relationship with others anxious and worried about our state of being? What if we are not so well, perhaps we would expend too much energy with learning to observe the senses and responses, energy that is maybe somewhere suggested as better spent on the healing processes, or alternatively we find ourselves in an environment that we know prevents us being able to utilise the senses and responses, you know a toxic one, but cannot get out of it, so cannot become aware of whether it is toxic or not, without the opportunity to observe response in an environment comparatively friendlier for these responses and our senses?

In consideration of how we ended up this way could it potentially be due to a general level of 'Societal Sensory Asphyxia', as consequence of being 'toxined-up', causing humanity's overall effectiveness in the X-system to have gradually compromised over the years, leading to further reduction in the ability to see and feel as clearly as we are capable in our environment? Add in a measure of mental fatigue theory from the Kaplans to be combined with this sensory asphyxia and one is at risk of generating a degree of 'Personal and Social Inertia', each being initiated by the other, existing as a result of a fatigue and lack of the energy needed to change the things we need to change in order to improve our world. A lack of sense combined with a lack of will is the possible outcome. It is difficult to say how long this has been going on for because it appears as to some degree as being virtually forever if looking at our history, and of course humanity is inconsistent in the potential of the X-system being accessed. However with the ways our living environment and lifestyles have fairly recently been evolving, and possibly for the worse regarding the introduction of a number of new materials potentially compromising to the senses, or should I say my own senses, there exists potential for a subsequent deleterious change to further cement the problem into a position in our lives.

So, could it be that society as a whole cannot see or sense so much generally, or is somewhat senseless, tired and apathetic? If people could really be able to see what's wrong are they lacking the energy and opportunity to act? Or maybe they could act but they cannot see what they should act upon? The end result is perhaps what we have, with many of the things we generally complain of in our society.

I'm not certain if I can make any sense of all this, what are the reasons for these phenomena existing? Surely our negative and positive responses have been necessary to best survive the world, it cannot be we have a design fault here, like our human Achilles heal, surely we are the most advanced model to have survived the tests of time? Or is this some sort of evolutionary quirk; a strength in our survival then becoming our weakness in further development?

Is it that when we don't have the capacity to act we don't see things in the same way as when we do have the capacity to act? Can it be we will then instead just operate on our reserve system until better times arrive again, and get by without using the senses because they are not accessible to us? One only needs to read the history books concerning our ancestors to learn of the hardships they had to survive for us to be here now. Through survival of the fittest, maybe as a result of all these hardships, humanity has possibly become hard wired to not see when it becomes more than we can take, and maybe as a species we have just evolved to survive and procreate without need of the senses. It almost seems that way, I mean we are regularly a bit dysfunctional or in denial of how things really are, or am I just speaking for myself here?

The local British Rail station adds for me a topic for reflection, concerning modern day planning and development. I'm sorry to say it, but what a grim, sad and sorry looking, uninspiring commuter hub this is to the greatest capital city in the world, host to the 2012 Olympic games. It is a joke yes? This 'greatest city in the world', is it just hype we are fed, or are we genuinely active in working to maintain the city of London's great reputation? Commuters could possibly arrive to this rail station refreshed from their homes for the morning trains and think, "What a dirty and unloved place, this should be improved", being my thought. It is possible these rail users may actually think this in the mornings. But then, after a day in the city, totally 'toxined-up', well that's me anyway and how I feel after this, hardly able to see my own hand in front of my face, or work out what I should get for dinner, let alone see all the things wrong with where I live and think of what action I should be planning to improve the way my world is for me. When I return home after my journey into town, the city, I'm beaten, I'm done, I'm broken. I think it could be the travelling more than the city itself, but I don't really know the source, possibly this is a package deal.

It's not so clear to easily see the beauty in things, or perhaps the need for it, when the senses and responses are compromised, the mind seems to become filled with words connected to problems and challenges to be resolved, clogging up the ability to sense and see. Is this why our world seems to obsess with things like the trains running on time 98.67% of the time, the functional considerations of our living environments and lives, because this is what happened, this is what we are still able to focus upon somehow whatever our condition, and even to two decimal places? Little doubt this is another evolutionary strength of man's.

Are the senses just becoming a luxury to be beneficially stimulated through our X-system in the modern world? It appears this way, present but obsolete to our daily requirement except for when concerned with nurturing of the arts or in the aesthetic appeal of nature and natural things. Is this state of things just going to progressively get worse and worse until we can just about see as far as the ends of our noses and work out how to put food we are given into our mouths?

Can we escape this living old before our time is due, or even living old at all? And is living more by our senses and responses going to be our solution to not only this matter of how we age, but also things like making more sustainable purchasing decisions, as Professor David Uzzell, of the Environmental Psychology Faculty at the University of Surrey, has been substantially funded to make his research upon? But we are quite possibly up against the odds, certainly in the short-term consideration, maybe always. Welcome to Shaun's fantasy world of the senses, remnant from some distant past era and fairy tales? Are we really too far gone to be able to wake up to what the senses have to inform us about, or in reality is it simply going to be way too complicated to facilitate a greater accommodation of the needs of our senses within our daily environment and way of life?

Visiting my local independent cinema the other day, showing a more art house type of movie, established a point on the dilemma to the sort of change that I might hope for. The decor of the cinema is tasteful, it has a carpet that suits me and allows my senses to flourish and appreciate what my now more open senses can take in of the movie's production. Yet I sit down and I'm itching about some how and realise there is something in my comfortable seat that is not agreeing with me, some material, who knows what, and on testing myself whilst sitting as compared to a later test when standing, my ability to inhale with the diaphragm, my LAPD, when sitting is only half that of when standing, simply as a consequence of the material the seating is made. Do I want to think about these things when trying to relax at the cinema? Not really, I just want to chill and enjoy the movie. But would I subconsciously have a better movie moment if the seating agreed with my responses or if I had not bothered to check the seating out in either scenario?

I am aware, to some extent, of how my X-system is influenced by my material world so I dress accordingly. I refuse to wear anything that compromises my senses and responses, even at the embarrassment of my wife, for instance if I'm wearing no underpants (due to the Elastin they contain and I personally do not respond well to). The problem my cinema example demonstrates is two fold. Firstly, I can change for myself but if I'm the only one cranky enough to dress for the reasons I do, why should the designer and specifier care about the X-system? It's a public place and business, they need to make a profit. Second, if we are wearing any material compromising to our X-system, then I do not think it will much compromise us further if we come into contact with it in the cinema, or other public place, unless of course we walk on it, possibly making it unsettle or agitate the X-system further through some sort of lack of 'earthing' phenomena that may be occurring. If we wear toxic we cannot spot toxic, we become blind to it's effects and the effects of other materials similarly affecting our systems. If we have a diet that compromises our system as well, you know we really have to forget the whole matter of the senses and responses, unless we actually starve ourselves for a bit, allowing our digestive systems to become refreshed. I think alimentary tract refreshment can even occur to some extent within a few hours, so that is at least helpful here.

The issue here is on how the world dresses, and if we dress poorly for the benefit of our senses and responses why should the world of interior design change towards the senses, other than to be more aesthetic or sustainable? Here again, another source to the stagnation of change, it's multi-level. Equally could designers be able to consider such matters without an appreciation and first hand knowledge of the X-system?

However, I do see so many instances in the use of materials in design where something is added to a product rendering it unfriendly to my own senses, which so easily need not be there and be quite easily replaced by something else potentially more response friendly at no more cost or even any loss in function. I guess this is the area of consideration where decisions can be taken at this early stage of making any change towards the senses, and as a supplement to designing products using more sustainable materials in their construction, even though I am not entirely certain on what 'sustainable' is completely about. I do know it's often a lot of head based thinking stuff, which I am somewhat against, and do not feel so sustainable in itself. In using the head to think and calculate too much it ties up the senses and responses, if we are not careful, a risk if this is what making more sustainable decisions comes down to, well possibly.

On a positive front, going sustainable and more natural in the past used to be to some extent a matter of altruistic choice on behalf of the consumer, no different to going organic in one's purchasing decision, where one is not sure if paying more will provide more than a feel good benefit for having performed or supported something positive. The senses and responses for me are supporting to the processes of going natural or green, and in choosing the potentially more sustainable option, for the reason of good health and a lot more potential benefit presently unknown to us. Could using the senses and responses become the new sustainable way of making green decisions, by way of us becoming more in tune with ourselves, and somehow we are naturally more tuned in than we might have imagined to the concept of us being sustainable within our character or make up?

No mass body of individuals I've at least heard of live, and are fully engaged, in today's world according to the senses and responses. There are many though still living more naturally around; perhaps traditional practising Mormons or the Amish who don't use synthetic materials as a part of their religion, and still use the horse and cart, but I'm not sure, or traditional peoples who continue to live by traditional means, or isolated communes in Europe cutting themselves off to some extent from the regular world to live more naturally, the likes of such being present within a few communities following the philosophies of Rudolf Steiner through Anphroposophy, as one instance.

Does it require cutting ourselves off to become more pure, or is it possible to fully engage in the world of today and still be able to utilise the senses and responses? So there's no research data or evidence in support of this approach to assisting decision making in our lives, which in a way is kind of cool really, if one thinks about it. Isn't there a bit of business opportunity here somehow, especially if it is as beneficial to mankind's future as it's appearing to me? Honestly, the senses and responses are potentially the basis to fuel the next Industrial Revolution, and double up as a means towards man's general evolution to being a bit more worldly savvy, turn humanity around in the current we are caught up in, knock down the recently built before the cement has dried too hard? Or will those interested in living by the senses just have to go find or establish hidden mountain valley or forest communities to live within?

Yet we do continue to live in an era with grand potential for false economy in our world's design, from the view of where the senses and responses are concerned. Making decision based purely upon functional benefits, aesthetics, reasons of convenience, savings of time and cost, for instance in building renovations, without considering the impact upon the senses and responses, provides this case example. Do people notice the difference if there is a synthetic timber simulate laid on the floor of a public restaurant and dining area, to cover the former worn looking original natural wooden and stone flooring surfaces, for instance at ones local stately home? Does this affect their repeat business and profits from receiving visitors? It could be the sales improve with the simulated timber flooring, but who's to say this wasn't as a result of the other general improvements made at the same time as those of the flooring renovations? It makes a lot of sense to lay the simulated natural material; cheaper and quicker to lay, possibly less down time for renovation and is easier to maintain, whilst still looking natural in appearance. This happened recently for me at the Hampton Court Palace, the former seat for Royalty in England. I was somewhat disappointed that the nice natural floorings of wood strip and old terrazzo tiles I had been used to in their cafe restaurant, albeit looking a bit worn and in need of attention, became covered over with plastic timber simulate during the restaurant's renovation, and I question if this a false or genuine economy that is being made here? Here is a place of national heritage, so surely money is no object?

I ask the question of whether the restaurant would have served more dishes with a natural floor, for instance if the former old flooring surfaces had been repaired and renovated instead or being replaced by being covered over with the timber simulate. Could the original flooring have potentially exerted a more positive impact on the X-system for the visitor, as a consequence would the food served have then tasted better perhaps with the old floor, would patrons stay longer without realising, eat a desert or have another drink? Would the kitchen chef's be more switched on and be able to tune in to what they were preparing, providing a greater opportunity for the food being potentially better received and agreeable to the senses and responses of the patrons and therefore more greatly enjoyed, or the kitchen chefs work in such a way as to reduce wasted food? Would staff manning the operation generally be happier, more charming and obliging to each other and customers, would managers be able to manage better, and the staff need less direction to do the jobs required of them? Would patrons feel more encouraged to make the return visit? Would a general subconscious feel good exist, with a financially beneficial twist, unassumingly hidden away in there as an added benefit simply from the flooring surface of the restaurant in question being made from a natural material?

Would people realise the prospective benefits of a natural flooring, over simulated natural looking surface, if wearing synthetic soled shoes? Ah, there's a good question. Where are the pitfalls and holes in all this, this hypothetical experiment for perhaps unravelling the benefits of creating environments more favourable for applying the senses and responses? And to make this thoroughly more complex, what if either material was fitted or finished with other materials compromising to the senses and responses of some or all of the users of the building? As there are many variables to be considered in this, would it help if everyone were to strip naked before entering the dining area, alternatively being dressed in the natural robes provided by the restaurant for the fullest sensory experience? Not here at today's Hampton Court, but I can strangely visualise something of this concept at a chic establishment for the super rich, however what about for the every day man and woman?

My own fantasy restaurants are to be found though, in the traditional regions of Europe as well as all around the world. Dirt floors or natural floors and natural surroundings, basic fare from the farm or region, I've eaten at them and it did excite me on every occasion, although I probably should not have drunk the farm made hooch they served when it was on offer. Fond memories. Yes, these places do exist, but often they are the novelties that time has over looked without a question.

My time is up, the Grim Reaper is heading my way so that's about all of it, as I now sit on the District Line, underground rail service into the centre of London this morning. I observe the variety in my fellow commuters to the city centre, although this for me is a one off trip and not the daily ordeal. More and more get on as the train makes it's way on and into the thick of the developed world, "oxymoron" I say to myself.

Many hold their hand held micro-processors in the form of mobile communication, work and reading devises. Is this the world for us, our future, this just the beginning of how things are to be? We can stay in constant communication, it is pretty incredible but do not our minds need to break? Do people read more or less with these new electronic tablet books, and what's the effect of these on the user and to the rest of us sitting here cooped up like cattle moving between farms, shoulder by shoulder, we are tightly squeezing in together.

People either side of me are wearing clothing that I know will be disagreeable to me, our legs and shoulders cannot help touching, unavoidable. It is like being a non-smoker near a tobacco smoker, but hey there's justice for the smoker this time, me, so who am I to complain of such situation.

I recall an old fashioned expression, "Don't bother trying to fix it if it ain't broke". Our society works, we feed ourselves and conduct our business, have healthcare, roofs over our heads, provision for children's education and old age, or sickness for when we have the need. All these people I am cringing about sitting next to, with their mobile networks and synthetic jackets, will earn substantially more than I, and I'm guessing have all these regular matters of society better planned and organised than in my case, especially on the financial provisions for old age. I have no real foundation or evidence to pass comment or judgement on the world supported by those I travel with on this morning's train.

In practise our world really does work amazingly. If we have an accident or develop illness our hospitals, doctors and nurses literally perform miracles in

Shaun M Sutton

keeping us well and alive, whereas in old times we would not have survived. Those I sit with make it work in spite of the clothing, diet, transportation means, homes and offices that I would estimate are not beneficial for using the senses and responses. These people around me are the genuine living testament to the system we have running it all as working and possibly, as compared with me, they are superhuman.

I feel myself foolish sitting here whilst on the train to the city to even dare consider anything else than what we have as working. In the back of my mind is a voice, distant, somewhere clinging on to be heard. A fog comes over me, I'm numb to the potential of life, the voice of reason has faded, just as the light has faded when the train went underground.

Feelings of the opportunity life holds and my senses in playing their part exist no more. Here is not a place to consider life's bounty or potential. That we can and do survive this all is demonstration of the strength of our system's we've created and our immune systems to survive these ordeals, evolved through centuries of men and women surviving repeated cataclysm, our ancestors.

The distant voice shouts, I just hear. "Don't take notice of what you think here, our world operates the way it does because of these places and ways, not in spite of". There's more, it's very faint and hard to hear whilst the train now sits at the Temple tube station. "The world in all it's ways would change if we live more to the senses and responses. Are we ready for this, can man ever be ready for this, will we always have two systems of operation, that for the senses and that for when the senses are compromised? At the moment the world operates according to the needs of the compromised sense, and that needs to change". I think I'm repeating myself now. I look at the faces on the train, we all look pretty tired, me too I guess, I feel it.

Notes

1- I took this quote from my own diary as having come from the Kaplans, but I now cannot find that quote and believe it might not come from their book 'The Experience of Nature', but is actually from another of their books, 'Cognition and Environment, Functioning in an Uncertain World', also published Ulrich's Bookstore, Ann Arbor, 1981, but I cannot presently find the reference I have made here.

World without words

How could we live in a world without words?
How would it work,
and how would we start to be mute?

"How is the weather?", "is granny better?", "my boyfriend's a rat!",
"my boss in an arse",
Expressions of life, of sorrow and joy, that are words.

Given our age of communicative bliss,
we live twenty-four seven should we wish.
A walk in the park, a trip to the sea, floating in a boat.
Where ever we are, words are on tap.

"Pour me a pint of you finest prose my dear!"
Sparkling clear, light amber hue,
filling my mind, life is a blast.
Mobile technology, love it or not, it's now in our blood.

What about quiet, when so much said and done,
starved of our thoughts, asphixiation by choice.
Loose sight of our dreams, motives and reason to be?

How to describe a scene in deep forest?
Sun shady glade, we've gone astray.
Grass under toe, a perfect blue sky overhead.

Infinite detail, colours brown blue and green.
Beat of a wing, sprouting of leaf.
The wafts of fresh cookies, but from where, I do not know.

Drawn into the wood, over grown and over run.
How long has it been?
Scratch my wings with back legs,
soak up the sun on my back.

Up and away, seek chocolate ice.
As I skirt about about bushes, then dance near the top of the trees.
What is chocolate ice?
I haven't a clue. Buzz, away and I'm gone.
I'm a fly.

In the park, Summer 2012

A guide on refining the senses to navigate the world of materials

-to go sense and response friendly-

Appendices 1-8

'The right leg'

Appendix 1 - Testing with the pulses -

How to perform the green moment pulse taking experiment

Within the texts of traditional oriental medicine discussing pulse taking as a means to assist in diagnosing the human condition, it is indicated that the physical and mental state of the physician are very important when feeling the pulse. The physician should be quiet, relaxed, and have the mind clear of other matters.

At the time of my original green moment pulse taking experiment I admit to not being completely clear on this point, unaware of a significance back then. I still struggle with finding the quiet mind state, it is perhaps less easy for me to find as it is to describe, although I commonly struggle with my grammar in the written word.

This experiment of my own fashion being described will hopefully help teach something of pulse taking through one's own observation, as well as in gaining some insight into what the sought after calm mind state actually is, and how the mind has influence upon the pulse. Grasping an appreciation of the mind's influence here is necessary in making any objective assessments by way of the pulse and other responses associated with the X-system, the mind needing to be as fully engaged with the senses as is achievable, and in trying not to think so much, or at least making an effort in this direction when there is a need to response test something.

This is the pulse taking method I still use to check my own responses to the various things in my environment. The description uses the example of testing one's pulse responses according to what is being thought. I refer to this as the green moment pulse taking experiment because when I first conducted the test I was staring out of the window to a garden area whilst monitoring the changes in my pulse according to what I was thinking upon.

The influence of the green, of nature, perhaps heightens the observations possible through nature's restful and restorative impact on our condition, as well as being encouraging to locating this more neutral mind state necessary to perform any response test. However, you don't have to stare out of a window at nature every time to response test, but if observing changes during response testing is found to be difficult, nature could assist if it is available to you.

The green moment pulse taking experiment

Sit comfortably facing nature. (I was initially looking out of the window, you could even be outdoors. Whilst this will influence the test as compared to being indoors, you should still be able to notice the way your pulse changes with the thoughts).

Find a comfortable posture that allows you to breath evenly in a relaxed fashion. Lightly place the finger pads of one hand onto the wrist at the radial pulse taking position of the other hand, located as per figure 1.

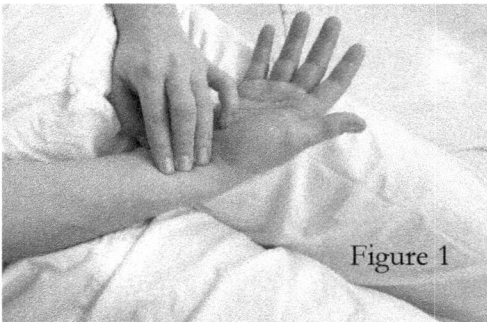

Figure 1
Where to locate the radial pulse for response testing

Notes to Figure 1
In order to locate the exact place for taking the radial pulse, bend the wrist so that the hand comes towards you, this makes an angle at the wrist joint. Place the ring finger of the other hand in the angle formed in the bend, on the radial pulse. Then straighten the wrist so it is more open and relaxed, resting the three middle fingers next to each other as shown in figure 1. Press each of the three middle fingers independently up and down so each is located directly on top of the pulse.

Lift up your head, adjust your posture to be comfortable, consciously relax the shoulders and take a couple of good breaths using the diaphragm. Let your arms relax and elbows fall at your sides whilst still holding the fingers in the radial pulse taking position, although your arms could be resting upon a table. Be mindful of muscle tension to support the arms and consciously minimise this.

Find the pulsation of the radial artery of the wrist. If it is not possible to feel the radial pulse of the wrist due to accident or injury, the test can to a certain extent be made whilst taking the pulse anywhere it can be felt, such as at the temples or just above the jaw by the ear canal, as shown in figures 2 and 3, where just two fingers are used.

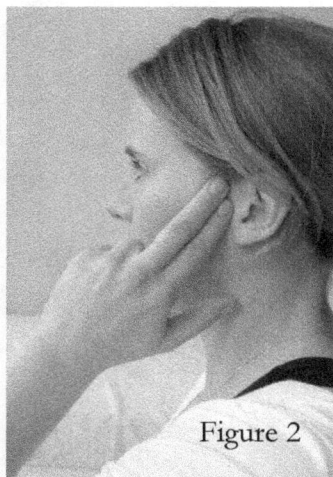

Figure 2

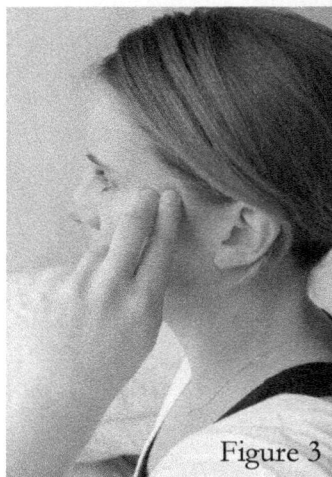

Figure 3

Figure 2
Where to locate the pulse at the ear

Figure 3
Where to locate the pulse at the temple

If it is possible for you to take the pulse on the wrist, roll the middle three fingers over the pulse and back a little at the location as shown in figure 1, in order to locate the place on that part of the wrist where the pulsation is felt at it's strongest, that is the place you need to be at. If you cannot feel a good clear pulsation but can just feel a very faint pulse, see if you can breath more with the diaphragm and allow the body to relax muscle tensions a little further. Sometimes it is necessary to search for the pulse a little deeper below the surface of the skin. Everyone's pulses are different, plus the pulse strength and depth are liable to change somewhat each day, and one side commonly has a pulse stronger than the other.

If the pulse is still just barely detectable, or hard to clearly make out, you can do one of two things. First, try taking the pulse of the other arm, so the test is made on the wrist that has the stronger pulse, making it clearer to observe any change during the experiment. Alternatively, if that does not help then read appendices 3 and 4 to ensure you are effectively using the diaphragm with which to breath, as this can strengthen the pulse and help it be clearer to read.

What you are aiming to piece together is a mental 2D or 3D image of how the pulse is appearing to you, in your own view, as in this test there is no right or wrong way in how you view it for yourself, it is for your information only.

Once you have located the place where the pulses are feeling at their strongest and most accessible, gently push the middle finger directly down into and then through the pulsing if you can, pressing as deep as is comfortable without increasing the pressure, and not pressing so much that you can feel the bone.

You will feel one of two likely scenarios upon gradually and gently pushing against the pulsing. The first is that you will be able to push through the pulse, so that the pulsing is no longer felt directly under the finger pad, and is now felt somewhat at the sides of the finger pad. The less common alternative you may find is that when pressed the pulse did not go away and you did not feel able to push through it, instead it was a feeling as though the pulse was pushing back against your pressure.

To then gauge the depth of the pulse from the surface, after locating the pulsing, ever so gradually lift the middle finger whilst still maintaining contact between that finger and the skin, raising it up until you can just about feel the pulse under the finger pad and then continue in raising the finger up towards the surface until you feel the pulse no more. To get a sense of how far the pulse is from the very surface of the skin, continue to lift the finger up until you are at the very surface of the skin above the pulse at that point where about to disconnect from the skin. You may or may not have possibly felt the pulse at the very surface of the skin.

Repeat the process of pressing the finger down and raising it up again to the surface of the skin to confirm or make clear the image in your mind of what you have been feeling. Also try to get a sense of the strength of the pulse, and size or width when you press on it, or for any apparent lack of force or size to the pulse being felt under the finger during this. The part of the finger you need to be using is the same as that which would be touching the thumb if you press the finger to it, at the finger tip.

Count the number of beats per minute, or this may be easier as beats every 15 seconds, or just get a sense for the rate of the beating rhythm, as it is the sense of something that may be easier to work with.

Here is a summary of what to look for in the pulse to assist in creating your mind's image of the pulse character for the purpose of this experiment;

• the distance between the pulsing surface and the skin surface
• the distance between the pulse and close to the bone
• the force or size of the pulse under the finger tip
• the general rhythm of the pulse's beating

As general information, under each of the three fingers there is commonly a different pulse picture , but for the purposes of this test just use the middle finger to create your own picture of the pulse during these early stages of obseving changes the pulse. Do not worry if you cannot get an image, just move onto the next part of this experiment.

Now focus away from the pulse and onto what is in your environment around you, using all the senses available to you to read the finer details of your immediate environment. Remain impassive to anything else other than what it is you can sense or see from where you are. Keep your eyes open, do not close them.

Here with a check list of what to consider in order to observe the most from testing anything with the pulses:

• the most ideal posture is the one that encourages the easiest and fullest diaphragmic breath

• allow the shoulders to drop and remain relaxed, and continue to check on this as you go

• adjust your posture regularly as you go to what feels the most relaxed

• breath rhythmically with the diaphragm, comfortably without feeling as though you are forcing the breath.

• loose all mental distractions, now is not their time and place, focus on feeling for and in forming an impression about your pulse's character, whilst remaining open to sensing the immediate environment.

• explore the finer points of your environment using all your available senses.

If the pulse character has been changing as you go, continue the exercise until there is no more change. The time to stop is the point when you feel you have something of an impression for yourself of the pulse whilst investigating your environment with the senses and noticing what is about you. That has now generated your green moment pulse picture if you have been exposed to nature, or alternatively your pulse picture for the hopefully now more neutral or impassive mind state generated when applying the senses.

Now switch your thoughts. Try thinking of different topics to see how thinking of these changes your pulse character from that of the green moment. Pick a topic, any topic and see how well you can get into the emotion of it, forget the impassive and actively engage the mind, whilst continuing to monitor any image you have for of the pulse, pressing gently down and slowly raising the finger up again until the pulse cannot be felt, and repeat. It could be reliving an experience, good or bad, but it is your test of how these situations and their related emotions influence your pulse that's all, nothing more.

When I did my original test, when thinking as opposed to sensing, I started off by thinking upon my overdue tax accounts and all the admin I was behind on, that got my pulses racing, these matters always seemed to stress me. If you don't know what to think of, then think of the tasks you have been putting off because you don't enjoy them, that should help to do the trick. Hopefully you should have managed to not have been thinking of these things too much whilst earlier seeking the green moment, but if you were, then you were, and this just means you will not notice such a difference between your pulse character for the different emotional situations.

Focus fully on just what you have chosen as a subject, don't wander from the emotion of the topic, observing the pulse as you go. If the pulse has been changing, and this in a way should have been fairly instant if you got into your topic, you can stop at the point where you have clearly identified for yourself that the pulse character has changed from that of the green moment for that emotional scenario, you should not try to torture yourself with it, this is just about identifying the pulse character changing according to your mind's focus. My recommendation is to not pick anything too traumatic to contemplate upon if you can help what you are thinking about. If you find you are able to mentally log each situation's pulse character, before again changing your topic of contemplation, by all means do so, but it's not really necessary. All one is aiming to achieve is to observe how the pulse can change from that of the green moment.

Once you have explored the pulse of your more active mind, then you need to return to the impassive and what your senses are relaying from the outside world, once more immersing yourself within the nature of your environment, go back to your original green moment, where the senses are doing the more active engagement in you, whilst still continuing to feel for the image of the pulse's character, pressing gently down and releasing, following the rhythm and beat. The exercise is not completed until you have explored something of the environment beyond yourself and things on your mind. This is no time to think about anything else, not even what's for dinner, or any other pressing or urgent matter you may have on for after your test.

If I had have drunk a coffee, smoked a cigarette, eaten a chocolate brownie or had any other sugary fix fairly soon before this experiment, I would be having difficulty properly exploring the place beyond the thought and engaging the senses to my environment. This materialises as any changes in the pulse during the test being less obvious, my system being overly drugged by these common stimulants, getting my pulse pumping. I would have difficulty finding the impassive state, but that's me, sometimes it is really not so easy to find the impassive and neutral mind state. If this becomes the case for you, try making the test in the morning before you have eaten or smoked or drunk, not even a tea, or herbal tea, just have some water if you are thirsty. Then you can be more sure of your mind not being too much under the influence of anything other than yourself. If you take medication in the mornings, try out taking it after the test if that can work safely for you just this time.

The most important matter during this test is to breath evenly and comfortably, and to not let the breathing stop by holding your breath whilst contemplating the pulse, or the breathing becoming shallow. If it is difficult to calm the mind and to only notice a slight or no difference between the pulse images during this exercise, in spite of having followed the advice given, it is best to focus on improving your skill and ability in using the diaphragm with which to breath. Putting the focus on developing the breath is always the most important of all things to remember.

However, if you have exhausted all the approaches mentioned here, including working with the breath as discussed in the other appendices, and remain having difficulty in observing any influence of your mind upon the pulses, you can check on the following.

The space you are in is completely quiet, no music, no TV, no phone, no computer, no talking.
Your pockets are empty, you have on no watch or jewlery.
You test on an empty stomach, drinking nothing but water, not even herbal tea.
You are not sitting within 1.5 metre / 5 feet from a bulk of metal or an electrical item, including lighting source or radiator.
You are not drunk or under the influence of recreational drugs.

If still it is not possible to observe any changes in the pulses, you could try taking off all your cloths and sit or stand wrapped in a big 100% pure cotton towel. The neighbours may begin to wonder about you if you sit at the window apparently staring at nothing, completely naked.

If you are still unable to observe any pulse changes in line with the thoughts, there is no need to feel disparaged. Study and practise the sections on how to breath with the diaphragm, keep practising some exercises for assisting in this at least once a day, twice is good if you are able to make the time, it need not take more than a couple of minutes if that is all you have spare, so it is really more of a matter of discipline than anything else. Alternatively be sure you include diaphragmic breathing within any regular exercise. You can try taking your pulse reading before you do your exercises and then again after to see if you can identify a difference between the before and after exercise pulse characters.

Learning to feel and observe for an obvious change in the pulse response may take time, it took me a few years to reach this point, so if you can get it straight away, well that will be quite exciting and an encouragement for trying to use and understand working with the senses and responses. Maybe you will just get it straight way.

Appendix 2

How to response test your trousers using the breath

Through beginning with sorting out the trousers, or in other words our basic and essential articles of clothing, to be more sense and response friendly, it is then clearer to identify our responses to other things we come into contact with. Also, the means described here to test the trousers is not much different to testing anything else. The benefit in starting with the most basic clothing articles is to ensure these are not influencing the responses before even beginning to test anything else, as opposed to these items potentially, and unknowingly, clouding the responses during testing to some degree. Above all, by beginning with the trousers it provides something to wear for when testing anything else.

In my original tests of clothing articles, at the time I had thought it necessary to wear them to test them, testing was then a bit of an ordeal with taking cloths off and then putting them back on. But at that time I was interested in appreciating the overall influence of the metals or other fastenings in them. Now I tend to perform the test by just touching the fabric of clothing, bearing in mind there may be different types of material used within various parts of a garment.

To allow for comparative testing with the breath, I use a scale by which to measure the capacity of my breath when testing, which I refer to as the 'diaphragmic inhalation count time', or DICT for short, which is the same as what I have also referred to as the LAPD within the tale of 'Trousers'. Once you can breath with the diaphragm this then provides a means by which to gauge the response on this and that being tested. The count is made in one's mind, at the approximate rate of one count per second, during one long smooth inhalation whilst only engaging the diaphragm to inhale. There is no inhalation count is not made for breathing with the chest, being the rib area, which should not raise when performing this inhalation count test. Just one continuous diaphragmic inhalation. The count is complete at that point of a genuine and obvious faltering, without engaging of the rib cage, to continue inhalation. The count at that point provides the measure for this particular response test, referred to here as the DICT.

A lower DICT when testing something, lower than it was before testing that something, indicates a compromising to the body organism, a higher count indicates some level of therapeutic gain should be potentially possible from whatever is being tested. And no change in the DICT means it is neutral to you at that time and place. It is possible that the responses can change over time for something being tested, or always provide the same response. It needs to be especially remembered with clothing, and occasional other things being tested, that if you are wearing or in contact with a material that is compromising to the responses without your realising, you will test something to appear as being neutral, but in actual fact it is not neutral, your responses were already being compromised by it before and during the test. This is why it is important to begin creating a response friendly wardrobe to wear in order to go around testing other things, especially clothing.

Here are a few extra notes on the subject of testing with the breath, in compliment to the key points detailed above.

Before discussing the diaphragmic response testing process, the most important of matters is to be consistent in how one inhales to facilitate testing. The key to performing the test lies in the art of using just the diaphragm to breath, or more accurately to inhale. This is indeed an art, one needs to consciously think about and apply oneself in using the diaphragm as a means for inhalation, and this requires more skill than may be imagined. For reason I do not understand, diaphragmic breath in many cases does not seem to naturally happen, either unconsciously or consciously, on its own. In general it seems necessary for it to be trained, with a few people just getting how to do it automatically and unconsciously. In reality the optimal diaphragmic breath comes when one is at one's most comfortable condition, and when one becomes most comfortable is provided for with the best diaphragmic breath. It is an art form coming out from the quality of the breath and body being reflections in the condition of each other.

Breathing with the diaphragm can be described very easily, or made very complex. However, whilst testing, one is trying to think as little as possible, so anything complex making has to be removed from one's mind. If you try to bear all these descriptions in mind, of the breath and diaphragm, you will find it harder to inhale whilst only using the diaphragm muscle, so whilst this is all maybe helpful to read it can also be unhelpful to bear in mind. Instead it is better to study the anatomy of the breath to facilitate a visualisation of breathing with the diaphragm, without thinking all about what it is you are doing in order to do it. Learn to feel how breathing with the diaphragm feels from your own experience. This allows it to be easier to think the desired 'nothing' when response testing using the breath.

I myself studied human anatomy many times, as a teenager at school on several occasions, then again in studying massage, then in herbs, then once again for acupuncture. Even after all these revision occasions somehow I ended up believing the diaphragm was located in the tummy, maybe somewhere around the tummy button, the navel. It was only some years after my studies were completed, when considering the subject more deeply, that it dawned upon me I had somehow imagined it wrong, even after all the years of study. Through a process of elimination I realised the diaphragm had to be higher up in my abdomen than I had earlier thought, in fact quite a lot higher. If you think you know exactly where it is and how it works, I recommend you double check it in anatomy books. (or alternatively in appendix 3, I have provided some alternative account of inhalation using the diaphragm) As for me, I admit to having been a very poor standard of student at the time of apparently learning about these things.

The breath test is no different to the pulse test of appendix 1, just one is counting in one's mind during a constant inhalation with the diaphragm, so everything applying to the pulse test also applies to the breath test. The specific benefit of the diaphragmic inhalation count time (DICT) test is that a number is obtained, a score to comparatively gauge things by, the count during diaphragmic inhalation. This is of greater value for comparative testing of different things and between different situations, where variable influences remain unchanged.

Performing the test

The difficulty with this test is that you cannot very easily stand in front of the window to make this test, as described in appendix 1 for the pulse test, but maybe you can stand far enough back so that nobody can see you from outside. If it's darker indoors than out, you may get away without being observed. So you need to remove all items of clothing, yes everything, removing all bracelets, jewels, trinkets, family air looms, stockings, socks and not forgetting all underwear. I once treated the mother of a regular patient, who had had all sorts of health issues over the years, whilst never once taking off her wedding band for about forty years, not once. At that time I was concerned over the potential influence of the wedding band on the condition of the physical body. Maybe its fine to leave certain things on, but how will you know until you have removed each of them and response tested for yourself with and without the item?

My feeling is that it is better to practice response testing with the breath when standing, which also improves the ability to test anything at a later stage where ever you are. However at this time you could sit, or lie on the floor if you prefer, especially if you do not want to be seen through the window. The flooring should be of wood or natural stone or another natural and unadulterated material. Carpeting can potentially be compromising upon the responses due to what it is made of or the underlay. Many floor coverings are as toxic to me as certain items of clothing, but you cannot be sure which are toxic to you yet. If you wish to, you can lie on a cotton towel on the natural floor, or wrap 100% pure cotton about you. I'm not sure what you would do if you think your whole living area has potentially toxic floor covering, but you may need to improvise. Don't move house or renovate just yet, it may turn out to test as being acceptable to your responses. Later, once you have assembled your best response friendly outfit, you can go out and test what you think of other places, and this way be able to work out what you think of your home, by way of comparing the DICT results for each location. I guess you could also lay or sit on a wooden table that is in contact with an emulsion painted or natural brick or unvarnished wooden wall structure, that would do if you were unsure of your response to the floor.

What is needed is your DICT whilst naked or wrapped in pure 100% cotton.

First exhale completely, to the point you cannot exhale further, then begin counting in your mind at the approximate count of one per second as you begin inhaling, just engaging the diaphragm. For me it seems to always be the same rate each time I make this inhalation test. When you reach the point, whilst inhaling, where you cannot further use the diaphragm to breath in, and the only way to inhale further is to begin engaging the ribs and upper body aspect of inhalation, then just stop, do not force it further, that point provides your DICT. It may start as low as 1 or 2, or zero, so don't be perturbed if this is the case, it just means you need to exercise and free up the diaphragm (see appendices 3 and 4).

Shaun M Sutton

The count rate is to a much slower inhalation speed than you may find usual. Inhalation can be done through the nose only or mouth. When engaging the diaphragm to inhale it somehow feels like you are breathing into the back of the throat when you have it correct, and in many instances makes a little noise as the air passes at the back of the throat, like a wind, appearing more so than in regular breathing. This noise used to irritate my wife in the early days, now she leaves me to it, but when hearing it knows I am testing something.

Exhalation is best done in a relaxed and controlled fashion, but the count for exhalation is unimportant in these tests. If you are finding it necessary to breath out, to exhale, much more quickly than inhaling, it is possible you could be forcing the inhalation more than you should and the count is actually lower than you thought. In which case re-do the test bearing this in mind, so that exhaling is more easy and controlled, and not like you are just coming up for air. After exhaling completely the test can be re-made. When the count is the same on two consecutive occasions, this provides your current naked inhalation potential (NIP in short), for how you are at that time and place. I use lots of names for the same thing so you can call it what you please. I thought NIP was quite a good one though, short for nippy or chilly, but acronyms are for fun and remembering the process.

I originally tried testing things with an inhalation count of about 5, although greater would have been more ideal to provide a higher degree of accuracy. Therefore the ideal NIP for testing clothing would be at least 7, in providing sufficient inhalation capacity to work with. Just test one thing at a time. As said you do not actually need to wear the item, but could hold it if allowing for different materials it may be made up from and test each of the materials separately, although if it has many different linings it may be worthwhile putting an item on.

To be sure of your response, the test should be repeated by taking a second inhalation, making a note of the count each time of the test. When you have two consecutive counts that are the same then take off the article or put in down, so you are no longer in contact with it. Repeat the NIP count test, as now the NIP may have increased through the exercise, in which case you need to re-do the NIP test again until getting two consecutive NIP counts that are the same as each other. If the difference between the NIP and count in contact with the clothing is just one or two (15-20% variation), this may not be indicative of anything. However be aware that you may have introduced a degree of sentimentality into the test by introducing the mind or desires, or really wanted a good result, because that tested was a favourite item, so you forced the breath to get a good result. The mind can easily play tricks to believe what is not so when testing. Keep sentimentality out of testing, stay neutral even if you don't think you could possibly live without an item you are testing in the wardrobe. I would be looking for a 30 percentage reduction in the DICT, when testing an article, as compared to the NIP to indicate a compromise. However, when starting out at this stage, a 30 percentage reduction may not be sufficient to be definitive, so check it again at a later time to see if the same thing happens or not.

When testing articles and finding something that actually does significantly compromise diaphragmic inhalation, through further testing it may be possible to observe what also happens with the pulse character, which would change in line with changes in the ability to inhale. This is of immense help in learning to understand what your pulse can feel like when the responses are compromised. This way one can teach oneself in how to read changes in the pulses and what they could signify within changes in the breath. Later you can notice other changes in you or in your perception through the senses, as there is in reality plenty of bodily responses to be observed when one makes oneself aware of these.

If there is something you find you are wearing that compromises the responses, but are unready to give it up just yet, as no alternative is available for you, remember you've been wearing it for a while without a care so do not worry about putting it on if you have to. However you need to remember it will be compromising your ability to response test and to notice a compromising from other items made of the same material. It then becomes necessary to seek out an alternative that performs the same functional job you require of that article, without a reduction in your ability to inhale with the diaphragm, it is as simple as that. The goal is to eventually be able to dress yourself in a completely response friendly outfit, and to see how that feels and how you then appear to the rest of world, without needing to remove all of your cloths to achieve this.

Recently I was able to obtain a pair of all leather sandals, leather sole and upper. I had been fantasising about this possibility for several years. Alternatives are out there, somewhere, sometimes to be discovered in some hidden lost world you may not be able to immediately locate, then all of a sudden you stumble across it. There may exist many old ways of doing things, using natural response friendly materials, that could be learnt from and response testing could be a way to help prevent certain skills becoming lost in the future. You could make your own if you are that way skilled. I remember making a pair of slippers from some odd carded wool off cuts I obtained from the company I bought my natural futon. They looked quite hideous, and did not take much skill to make, but they did the job of keeping my feet warm without having to compromise my responses, and only a few people had to witness my wearing of them. Surprisingly I also had fun making them.

Here are a few things that could limit diaphragmic inhalation;

*   All those things mentioned for the pulse taking test in appendix 1.
*   Distracting noises (even the kettle boiling puts me off my test).
*   Testing too many things in one session (set a limit of no more than 3-4 things to begin, increasing the number as confidence and ability improves).
*   Stressful days or being ill.
*   Being pressed on time.

If any of these above things are happening and you are getting confused with your testing but still have the need to test something, such as a remedy that may help out, then you need to triple test it if you are not sure (see appendix 7) rather than relying on a more standard double test. Make sure you are not relying on just the one way to response test, all the other possible tests should agree and confirm the same result. This way you can best avoid making error. If you are not sure about the response, this indicates an inconclusive test, so don't take anything from the test. If you are stressed, go read or do something else relaxing to calm the mind. You might be hungry for simple foods but fantasising junk. That is the state of being sick leading to thinking nonsense. Always aim at testing in your best condition, try not to be hungry, but be aware your food can compromise your responses.

When I'm ill my inhalation capacity can be down to half of even a third of what I would normally expect. If you find it possible to do something that causes an increase in the diaphragmic inhalation capacity, your health at that moment will improve somewhat. This can help in gaining a better understanding of how good and bad health feels, as well as observing other ways of gauging health, beyond the state of more obvious symptoms associated with an illness.

Once you have worked out how, breathing using the diaphragm is very easy, but do not be disappointed if you find it very difficult in the beginning. This suggests you really do need to work on it.

If you are not in a good place to make change, or are anxious about how your life could change as a direct result of better breathing with the diaphragm, then if you wish to try it out, just slowly integrate diaphragmic breathing into your life. Better breathing allows for clearer observation if you do test something. Wei-she, one of my oriental medicine teachers, once said to me, "change should be not too fast, if it's too fast it is not so good."

A couple of close people I know experienced panic attacks and palpitation when they first started breathing with the diaphragm, but it was just momentary and I have no real idea why that occurred.

I have to admit that I am currently adapting my diaphragmic inhalation response testing method, placing my focus more upon reading the smoothness and ease of the diaphragmic inhalation, as opposed to counting the time of the full inhalation. This makes testing quicker, so within a count of 10 or 15 I am aware if the response will at least be positive or negative. Also who knows, but at a later time it may be discovered that long term over working the diaphragm is bad for your health, I mean it is a bit unnatural, unless you are a pearl diver. Overall I think it is wise to explore a variety of response testing means, even try coming up with your own through careful observation of what else happens when the pulse and breath tests are showing a compromise or improvement, as part of the overall refinement in the use of senses and responses.

One extra test I now regularly add in is the 'neck turn test'. When the responses improve physical tensions in the body lessens which usually, but not always, includes relaxing of the neck and shoulder muscles, that is if they were tight. Currently I just use this for testing things more of a therapeutic value, but it is possible to use the test in inverse, as anything compromising the bodily responses would lead to a tighttenting of these muslces, with greater limitation in movement. When I perform this test I find it works best if I look along a book shelf to see which is the furthest title I can see, and then observe if this changes. This may help one appreciate how to create one's own personal test methods. The 'neck turn test' is my favourite double check test of my other testing methods.

For more on using of breath and other responses as a guide to health and in the treatment of illness further information is in appendix 7.

As the DICT increases over time, which it will with practice and from making changes to improve the responses, this refines the ability to test. There were things I tested earlier on that I thought where agreeable to my responses, yet in the back of my mind whenever I used them I felt some strange impression it was not quite right. Then on retesting them in the future, with my wider DICT scale, I found they were compromising my responses by a third. This is the difference just a count of 3 if the DICT, without the item, was 10, which is not such a margin for error. But then later this 30% difference could become almost 7, when my capacity to inhale with the diaphragm has increased to 20. When getting an odd feeling about something, just test again when you are in a good or better shape.

Here is an ancient quote about breathing, maybe it helps support bringing the significance of the breath and diaphragm into a broader view. I just recently came across it in the book 'Alchemy, Medicine & Religion in the China of A.D. 320', by Ko Hung, translated by James Ware, first published 1966 by the Massachusetts Institute of Technology. This quote is taken from Chapter 18. Theoretically this makes it about 1700 years old, although one would expect some loss of Ko Hung's original meaning through the centuries and translations, which will unavoidably have modernised the text.

"The body of an individual can be pictured as a state. The diaphragm may be compared with the palace, the arms and legs, with the suburbs and frontiers. The bones and joints are like the officials; the inner gods like a sovereign; the blood like the ministers of state; the breath like the population. To take good care of the population is the best way to make your state secure; by the same token, to nurture the breaths is the way to keep the body whole, for when the population scatters, the state goes to ruin; when the breaths are exhausted, the body dies. Anything that is dying cannot be living, and anything that is perishing cannot be in a state of preservation. Therefore, man in his highest form dissipates fears before they arise; he controls illness before it occurs. He does his doctoring before anything happens; he does not pursue what has already gone. Just as a population is hard to nurture but easy to endanger, so is it difficult to purify the breaths, but easy to soil them. Therefore, as a careful control of power is the way to protect a state, the way to strengthen the blood and breaths is to whittle down covetousness. After that, Truth-Unity survives, the three Hun and seven Po are preserved, all harm is dispelled, and life is extended."

(Hun and Po are the inner spirits/gods of an ancient Chinese conceptualisation for the living body)

Appendix 3

The anatomy and mechanics of a diaphragmic breath

My first experience of breathing with the diaphragm was what I would describe as belly breathing practiced in an early class to learn Qi gong, suprisingly in the former Eastern part of Germany, whilst visiting a friend. Having partnered ourselves up we took turns to have one person lie down face up, whilst the other gently encouraged that supine person's belly flat with the flat of their hand as they exhaled. Whilst the supine began to inhale, the partner tried to encourage the tummy to rise up to be as big as possible, lifting the flat of the hand upwards, maintaining contact with the belly, before again letting the hand follow the belly down with the exhalation. I did not have a clue what was supposed to be going on, they were only speaking in German, and at that time the Berlin Wall had only recently come down so not many people spoke any English in the Eastern region, and my German speaking was even more limited than it is now. As a result I really found it a very difficult exercise and felt I had embarrassed myself at how badly I did it when I was the one lying down doing the belly breathing. Honestly, they were almost laughing at how hopeless I was at it, I tried laughing too, how could such a simple looking thing be so difficult in practice? I mean, hello, I've been breathing since I was born, so what's the big deal here? I was too embarrassed and proud to even mention that I could not belly breath to the teacher, who was the friend I was visiting.

I come from humble diaphragmic breathing beginnings. A few years ago in Mexico, I was asked if I could treat one of the locals who worked where we were staying, and who had a persistent pain in his stomach. I spoke no Spanish and he no English. So I showed him how to breath via demonstration, inhaling with the diaphragm, my hands on my tummy to extenuate the degree my belly came out on inhalation, and the difference between the inhaled and exhaled belly states. I explained to him it was the Buddha breath, as all those little statues sitting in gardens of the Buddha depict him with a big healthy round belly, and as well near to our apartment there was a night club called the 'Buddha Bar'. Anyway, he seemed to easily get how to belly breath with this explanation and by the end of the session was breathing like a Buddha himself, plus his belly ache cleared up to make it appear as though I was some sort of miracle worker locally.

Over the years I have attempted all sorts of means to get across the importance of breathing and often despaired when a patient is struggling with making it, just unable to get it, their mind unaccustomed in how or why even to use it, how to begin, trying to do it but being unsuccessful. I think there had been times when it almost felt like I was torturing some of my patients with various ways to kick start them using the diaphragm when they were not able get it. It seems it is like being able to swim or ride a bicycle, once you've got it it is easy somehow, but when you haven't ever learnt, and especially when older it seems much harder, perhaps because we've got to overcome a lot more issues getting in the way of re-learning what we already know. Kids seem to be able to do it very easily via demonstration.

In my earlier practice I had been considering the functioning of the diaphragm from the way it is taught to us, being how we get air into our lungs, as a part of the whole respiration thing, I never genuinely understood it it, but once I started to consider the diaphragmic breath from another perspective, from the other side of the same coin, in the discrete functions and forgetting a more obvious role in respiration, being how we use oxygen, I was better able to appreciate it all. The secret is in thinking of the role in respiration as some sort of bye product of what else the diaphragm does, I think that's the best way to appreciate how it works and to consider wher the diaphragm is located to assist actually breathing with it. Taking out the diaphragm's considered role in respiration quite possibly makes it easier to understand the internal process going on. The big key for me was to consider what is located adjacent to the diaphragm, in fact directly under, by way of a group of the body's major blood filled organs.

Of course it is no whim of evolution that we are designed the way we are, with a significant group of internal organs, crucial to our body's function, sitting just below and in my mind adjacent to the diaphragm, we are a perfect design. Our kidneys, liver and spleen are all located in set positions, all protected from injury behind the ribs, and not forgetting the heart, sitting just below the centre of the chest. Again, to best understand the diaphragm's function one needs to put aside, just for a moment, it's classically considered purpose in life, of sucking air into the lungs to obtain oxygen and expel the waste products of respiration.

I mention all this because I was never able to assemble the whole thing, how we really functioned. When I learnt things we tended to learn each organ's function in isolation of the other parts. Maybe this was just me, and the way my learning brain worked was to think of each separately, the same way as I learnt to answer exam questions, and subsequently receiving my qualifications I was studying at.

It may already be clear I'm no anatomist. I virtually passed out during an anatomy lecture, one of examining some parts remaining of half a human body, to iden-tify this and that at Guys hospital in London. I used to bribe my anatomy lecturer with little presents earlier in the year to subconsciously prime him for being extra kind to me in the final oral test examinations, when I was already predicting I was going to fall apart. I suffer anatomiphobia. So if you really want to know how it all goes down, inside of us with the organs and breathing, I recommend you look it up from the accounts and diagrams of a professional anatomist, and that is not me.

What I can supply, as an alternative idea, is my own layman's impression of what I imagine is occurring, and from the consideration of the diaphragm in my lay-man language only. What I say is without doubt technically incorrect, so don't take it as fact. These ideas about the diaphragm are intended to just help me visualise in my own mind what it is I guess is going on, so as to be able use the diaphragm more appropriately during inhalation. Here's my own account.

"My ribs create a fixed bell shaped cage, which cannot move or flex. Towards the bottom of the cage, at the back, are the kidneys, each about fist size, to their right is the liver, the size of our two interlaced hands, to the left is the spleen, again fist size, and at the front is the heart. All these organs cannot be touched, they are hidden, protected behind the cage. The diaphragm sits directly on top of all these, inside the bell shaped cage. All these organs are loosely fixed in their places to stop them falling out of the cage and getting damaged.

Due to the need to squeeze a lot of organs into a small space and perform it's functions, it so happens that the diaphragm ended up curved concave, going further up in the middle of this cage. The diaphragm is then firmly fixed to the inside the perimeter of the cage, attaching to the lower ribs, and laying directly above each of all those internal organs, which are tightly squeezed in under it.

Above the diaphragm is loosely attached the lung tissue, in the upper part of the cage, within a kind of vacuum so that any movement within the cage affects the volume of air held in the lung tissue, which itself is formed like those old fashioned bath sponges.

The diaphragm itself is all muscle, it is a solid complete sheet of muscle, dividing the whole of the upper body from the lower body. When inhaling with the diaphragm all that is in fact happening is the diaphragm's muscle fibres are contracting, no differently to what happens to make a fist or flex the arm for instance, working by way of the muscle fibres becoming shorter through their contraction. As the cage is firm and fixed and cannot move, when this concave muscle sheet's fibres shorten the whole diaphragm gradually begins to flatten out, descending to press against all those organs squeezed in underneath it, to push them downwards in increments with each further contraction of the diaphragm muscle's fibres. It's a gradual bit by bit thing, it can only occur at one slow set speed. All the internal organs being pushed against take time to squeeze down, little by little, all their own connections that hold them in place having to stretch somewhat as it goes, all re-organising in position together.

On the other side of the body, the other side of this world of re-organisation, whilst all that activity is going on down below in the lower abdomen, above the diaphragm more space is being created in the vacuum upper half of the bell cage, causing the spongy lung tissue to be released like relaxing pressure off the bath sponge, which fills with air being automatically sucked in through the nose or mouth, and the lungs to simultaneously fill with the air from outside us.

Back to down below the diaphragm, where all this pushing and squeezing is going on, there is a knock on pushing, and like a crowd all pushing one way they have to go forwards. This forces the organs against the intestines and stomach, even upon the bladder and internal sex organs, they all get pressed against, as the diaphragm muscle fibres contract, and the sheet of the diaphragm muscle pushes against them all. There is only one way to go and that's out, out starts to pop the belly, little by little, not just at the front which is most obvious, but also to the sides and at the back to an almost equal extent, as the diaphragm continues to contract and squeeze against all the internal organs located just below it. As we do this, air is constantly being sucked in through the nose or mouth.

When we can no longer activate contraction of the diaphragm muscle, no more air is sucked in through the nostrils via activation of the diaphragm and no more the belly is displaced outwards."

For practicing diaphragmic breathing I'm not interested in anything more than this. Not why the belly pops out in the way it does, or what happens on exhalation, or where does everything shift to, or why is it that sometimes it's easy and other times it's just not working so well, or why is it that contraction seems to work at just one steady slow speed that I can seemingly have some control over. I've considered all these, but they are unimportant when making the diaphragmic inhalation. All one needs to appreciate is that at the end of exhalation, it can all begin again.

I have always had the idea all this internal squeezing going with diaphragmic inhalation must be like doing an internal massage of sorts, contributing to things working better on the inside of the abdomen, assisting all those main organs keep us alive, by working better, helping the blood flow more effectively through them. It's just a thought, I appreciate the living organism may be more complex than my mechanical view of its operation. If it helps encourage more use of the diaphragm, then the idea serves a purpose.

Whilst I inhale with the diaphragm, in order to test how it responds to my world, all I'm thinking about is hopefully nothing, none of any of this. All I am doing is feeling the diaphragm displacing the contents inside my lower abdomen, keeping my shoulders relaxed, posture upright, counting in my mind, looking around me or seeking to sense my outer world, my non verbal world, and to not think about anything at all, as much as I can.

Appendix 4

Exercises to help improve the ability to breath with the diaphragm

There exist all manner of professions, practitioners and hobbies that either encourage the use and exercise of the diaphragm muscle, or help in releasing a stuck diaphragm that has forgotten how to work, freeing it up somehow so it can operate better. Some of these may have a spiritual aspect attached, immediately thinking of Yoga, others think more mechanically, others of its practical benefits.

I personally think anything helping to stretch the body's connective tissues, especially around the lower abdomen, could be useful to the diaphragm's func-toin. For instance, my personal favourite exercise for stretching the connective tissues of the abdomen, in a way beneficial for using the diaphragm, is to go out blackberry picking in the hedgerows for an hour or so, but unfortunately that's only possible for a few weeks each year, and if we all went picking berries there would be fewer left for me. Maybe we should encourage brambles a bit more. It is outdoors, there is stretching the body in nice ways, it is calming and therefore therapeutic on the mind, it is what our bodies are naturally designed to do, and we get something else from the exercise beyond the exercise, so really it needs to be viewed as a much more sustainable a form of exercise as a result of several benefits coming from one activity. Maybe painting and decorating can have a similar effect, although I'm not sure about the effects of some of the paints on the responses, and it does not provide the outdoors or tasty berries.

One of the most outlandish inhalations I have ever witnessed was by a friend, laying on my therapy table, who was a Pilates teacher. Man that was crazy, I've never seen anything like it before or since. It was definitely very different to how I have described inhalation, but who's to say it was not just a more evolved and expert version of the diaphragmic breath? My breath may be the standard, but that was certainly the deluxe. All I can say, in support of my simple version, is that through its simplicity one can test, as there are fewer other variables to get in the way of making before and after test comparisons. However, perhaps this sort of elaborate training can help in freeing up the diaphragm in functioning, I'm sure it does help. It may be it is possible to work out one's own method of breathing in order to successfully response test at a future date.

I once observed a chap, a physiotherapist, exercising near me in the park, doing all these hip rolls and pumps and further contortions of the body. I asked him what he was doing and he told me he was engaging the diaphragm muscle. Some of my patients who are best able to breath with the diaphragm have been sports people and were trained to use it. Others have been singers or played wind instruments. I'm just thinking that swimming has to be good for the diaphragm, although again I'm not sure about the effect of the chlorine added into the water of our modern day swimming baths on the responses, perhaps one day there will be something potentially less toxic in replacement.

There are a lot of people actually using the diaphragm to breath, so for many it is just a short step to use it for testing one's environment. Plus, there are many enjoyable activities encouraging use and exercise of the diaphragm muscle.

A massage teacher I once studied with informed us that the body is one big interconnected mesh, like a woollen jumper, and if you pull one part it affects the rest. If you cannot exercise, but have some way in which you can move something, then move it and exercise what you can, to observe how your flexibility is linked with the way your diaphragm is operating, or not. I think this would make for an interesting exercise.

Another massage teacher suggested that in order to once again learn how to breath properly, where the diaphragm had become stuck or lazy, you had to first breath out, exhaling until you could breath out no more, then wait, wait until you really have to inhale, then inhale as far as you really can. I thought it a little extreme, but maybe that will help someone crack it and kick start the stuck system.

In an ideal world we should not consider this as just an exercise to be performed in isolation, that would be missing the point, ideally we should be outdoors. Yet if the weather does not allow one to get out, or if right now we cannot get out doors, or do not have access to further research in using the diaphragm, here is my own variation on the exact exercises that actually had me first consider how I was breathing, and started me off in using the diaphragm with which to breath.

These specific exercises have been adapted from those I first studied in the book 'Five Elements and Ten Stems - Nan Ching Theory, Diagnostics and Practise', by Kiiko Matsumoto and Stephen Birch, published 1983 by Paradigm.

Basic exercise to help breathing with the diaphragm

The basic exercise for inhaling and exhaling with the diaphragm is performed whilst lying on your back, with the knees bent, and feet resting on the surface you are lying upon, if possible, which could be a bed or a hard surface like the floor. If you place you hands on top of each other just over or below your tummy button, or what is technically named the umbilicus, when you are breathing into the belly by way of using the diaphragm the hands will naturally slide apart somewhat on inhalation, and slide back again on exhaling. I felt that observing this movement of the hands helpful when I began practicing this, as a form of awareness feedback means when using the diaphragm during inhalation. However, I have observed a few patients over the years who try to thrust out their tummy, by way of using muscles other than, giving the impression of inhaling with the diaphragm, but actually they were inhaling using the ribs of the chest and not the diaphragm. If you are unsure in using the diaphram, appendix 3 may help.

- Basic exercise for inhaling with the diaphragm.
referring to Figure 4

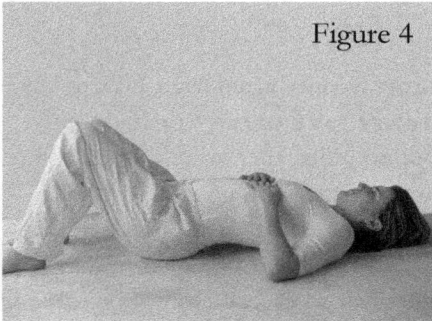
Figure 4

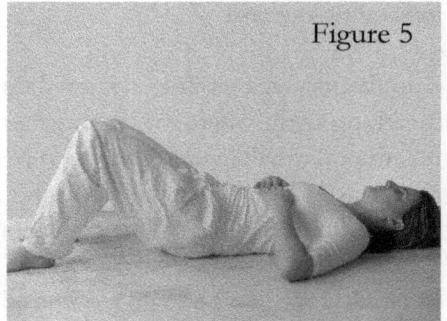
Figure 5

Whilst inhaling, the back is arching up a little so that the small of the back will possibly be lifting off of what you are lying upon, that is if you are quite flexible and what you are lying on is a hard surface. This occurs through the low back's muscles being tightened, using very gentle tension sufficient to arch the back in a comfortable and unforced fashion, and definitely avoiding any discomfort through forcing the arch. As a result of this, and inhaling with the whole of the diaphragm, a further stretching up and out of the low abdomen is achieved. Whilst you perform this part of the exercise count in your mind during the inhalation until you cannot inhale any further.

- Basic exercise for exhaling with the diaphragm.
referring to Figure 5

Whilst exhaling, the small of the back becomes pressed against what you are lying upon, as a result of the pelvis swivelling in the upward direction, so that the tailbone may even be lifting up a little. This does not involve any pushing up with the legs to lift the bottom up, just a light contraction of the deep muscles of the tummy. Just use very gentle tension sufficient for the back to no longer be arched, without forcing the movement or causing any discomfort. Count in your mind the exhalation, whilst doing this, until you cannot exhale any further. Then repeat the inhalation exercise, starting as at figure 4.

As an exercise to improve the control of the breath one aims at taking at least as long to exhale as it takes to inhale. The original exercises suggested taking twice as long to exhale as to inhale, but this depends on the speed of inhalation. The main issue is in controlling the exhalation, before inhaling again. When doing this exercise myself I find it necessary to think about nothing at all to acheive this, and find the performing the exercise as desribed .

Begin with five or ten rounds daily for a few days or weeks, gradually increasing to twenty inhalation and exhalation rounds if you are that way inclined, or continuing until it takes twice as long to comfortably exhale as it did to inhale, whilst experiencing a very much a full inhalation for you. (i.e. you could do much fewer rounds as you become more proficient in controlling the exhalation).

When I first started trying to exhale for twice as long as it took to inhale, I think I started at inhaling for a 5 count then exhaling for 10, just about. As one begins to inhale for a longer count, exhaling for double that requires calm mind, and in a way this probably compliments what is achieved from the exercise, by encouraging the mind to calm. The original exercise I learnt recommended exhaling to a count of 20.

The exercise can be adapted as one gains proficiency in it, and the movement performed during the exercise should be gradually made during the count, so that it flows more smoothly. I personally found it harder to perform this simple exercise than I had imagined. If you cannot lie down sitting can work to perform the exercise.

-Beginners exercise to help free up the diaphragm muscle
referring to Figures 6, 7 and 8.

This exercise is performed whilst lying on your back with your hands under your head and your heals as close to your bottom as you can comfortably get them, with your feet resting on the surface you are lying upon, which could be a bed or a hard surface, like the floor.

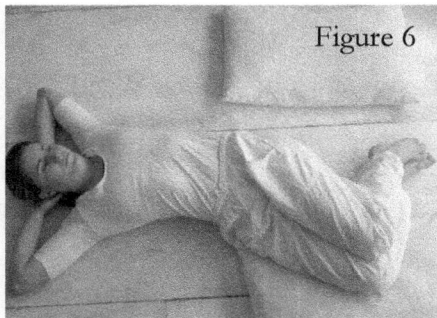

Figure 6

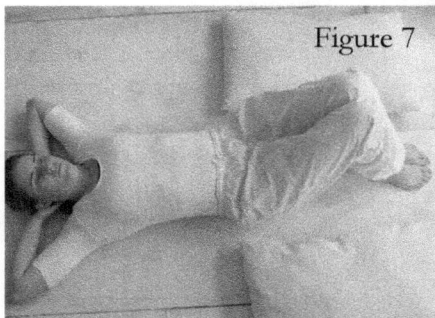

Figure 7

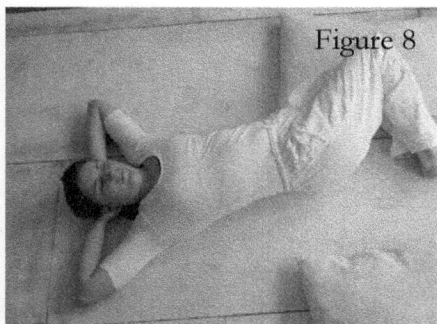

Figure 8

Figures 6 and 8
Knees swing to the left,or right, during the exhalation, ending to be supported by pillows.

Figure 7
Knees central until completing a full inhalation.

By positioning a pillow, or a stack of pillows, at each side of the body, this facilitates the hips being more able to fully relax when the legs are swung over to one side and then the other, without causing any discomfort during the exercise. If there is any potential for discomfort then increase the number of pillows, acting as a support at each side, until there are sufficient to easily make the exercise. You could even use a box at each side to rest the knees against, as long as it does not slide away. Remember to begin cautiously, especially if you are aware of an old injury, limitation or weakness. Only gradually reduce the number of pillows at your sides during, over days or weeks, to allow the body to adjust gradually, without risk of discomfort. Also should be aware that cushions and pillows are very often made using components compromising the breath, so check before using what are available, as described in appendix 3, otherwise benefit less will be achieved.

Perform the exercise slowly, in a controlled fashion, allowing the knees to swing to each side until they are resting comfortably against the pillows at the sides, whilst slowly exhaling until the knees have come to rest on the pillow supports. Inhale with the diaphragm whilst simultaneously bringing the knees up to the central position, having fully inhaled. Begin exhaling whilst allowing the knees to slowly swing to the other side, until they are resting comfortably against the pillow, fully exhaling. Then start inhaling with the diaphragm whilst bringing the knees to the central position, having fully inhaled, and repeat the exercise.

Begin with five to ten rounds for a few days, gradually increasing the inhalation and exhalation rounds as you feel more capable of doing so, or continuing until it takes twice as long to exhale as inhale, whilst experiencing a significantly full inhalation (you could perform fewer rounds when having mastered control of the exhalation). The exercise specifically helps in releasing or appreciating tension in the hips and abdomen whilst inhaling with the diaphragm, and to increase the inhalation capacity when using the diaphragm.

If you feel stiffness of the body after doing the exercise, perhaps you over did it, so either increase the number of pillows or reduce the number of rounds.

-Advanced exercise to help free up the diaphragm muscle
referring to Figures 9 to 12

This is an extension of the beginners exercise. Here the head turns in the opposite direction to the knees, and there is just a slight or no pause in the middle with the knees in the vertical central position, at the point of the inhalation reaching it's fullest capacity. Whilst figures 9-12 depict the hands resting under the head, one equally could spread the arms completely out at a 90 degree angle from the body, with the palms facing down for a further advancement of the stretch, or palms facing up for intermediate level work. Note the maximum exhalation occurs after the knees have completely swung to each side, and inhalation begins again before the knees are lifted off the ground.

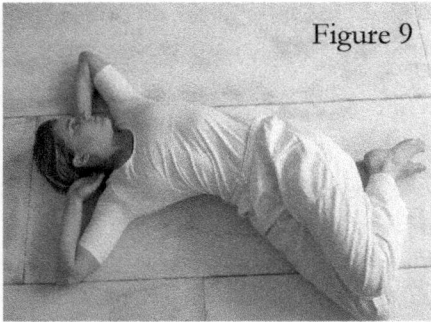

Figure 9
The point of full exhalation as the knee begins resting on the ground.

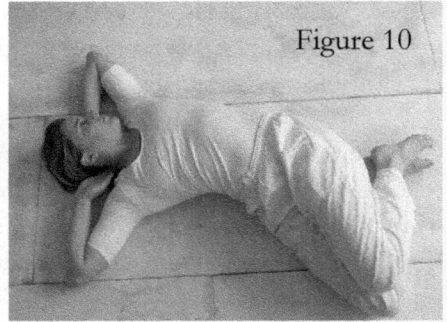

Figure 10
Beginning to inhale just before lifting the knees off the ground to swing them over to the other side.

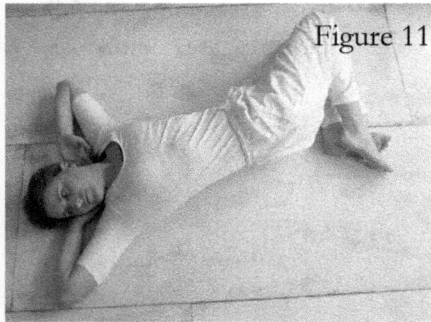

Figure 11
The point of full exhalation as the knee begins resting on the ground.

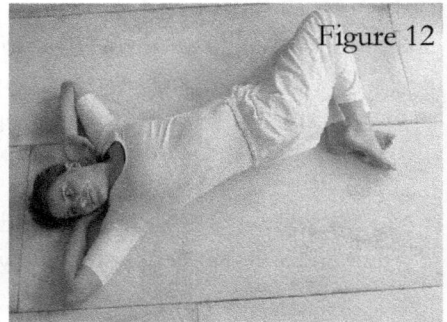

Figure 12
Beginning to inhale just before lifting the knees off the ground to swing them over to the other side.

Commence with the beginners exercise just in case you are not as flexible as you imagined, or used to be. The eventual aim is to keep as much of the back touching the floor as possible whilst keeping the heels fairly close to the bottom, but this is a later consideration. As ever work within ones comfort, never experience any pain or injury or forcing the exercise into a stretch. It is about 'allowing' the stretch to occur without discomfort of any form, at any stage.

Another adaptation I have practised of this exercise, for much later on, is to rest the foot on the knee during the swing over, but I am not sure much more is achieved other than adding to the risk of over stretching, so caution.

The number of rounds performed depends on what is wished from the exercise, but experiment in this, as it may be that after a certain number of rounds extra gain can occur. Potential for gain can be monitored through the pulse and breath, or other aspects observed as liking to the X-sensory response system. Monitoring the responses before and after exercise allows an assessment of what has been therapeutically gained. I would expect these particlar exercises described here can be performed in such way to be able to observe significant improvement in the X-system bodily responses. See appendix 5 for more thought on this topic.

Appendix 5

Linking any practice to the X-sensory response system

It should be considered, and maintained in mind, that the most advanced form of an exercise, or any practice, is likely that guided by way of feedback obtained from observing any aspect of the 'X-sensory response system' (the X-system).

These exercises or practices do not need to be very physical in nature, but can be anything requiring a special connection between the action and medium being worked with, such as in any art form, profession or practice where there is the potential for an improvement in the X-system, observable through the practice. This will probably be representative of a comparatively higher form of practice.

Learning how to make observation of the senses and bodily responses can as such provide assistance in guaging one's own development and progression within any particular practice, through reflection with these means of feedback.

Understanding something of the X-system supports a broader appreciation of why, and how, we practice what we do in life, as well a glimpsing, perhaps, of the truer personal goals to be aimed for within our practices.

Extending on from being able to master what we practice, onto our making of decisions, it feels to me as though the better decision is more likely where the senses and responses are being nourished and flourishing nearer their optimum. Conversely, there is a greater potential for poor quality decision, and consequent actions, when the senses and responses are compromised by the materials we use, our environment, and any illness or subsequent treatment we may be receiving.

Matters of health need to be viewd as just one of many symptoms associated with the workings of the X-system. Considering matters of toxicity only in terms of an influence upon health and illness limits one's ability to explore the costs associated, for instance, as a result of sub-optimal decisions and a consequent set of actions, if living with material environments compromising us in some way.

Working with the 'X-system' can as such liberate more limited views upon health.

Appendix 6

Debating healthcare with regards to the senses and responses

I am apprehensive about discussing the subject of healthcare, simply as this risks overly limiting consideration of the senses and responses to a health perspective.

To me matters of healthcare are a taboo subject for discussion when in polite company, more so even than those of religion or politics, simply because everyone holds their own beliefs on this subject, by which they potentially order their lives around, and not everyone shares the same beliefs. One could contend that the subject of 'how to stay alive and well' is about as serious an issue as one finds, more so than those of politics or religion, being themselves merely extensions on from the healthcare agenda. Differing beliefs on healthcare can easily lead to heatedly contentious viewpoints. I'm just thinking upon the sorts of discussion, or should I say argument, I shared with my German parents in law about such things to be reminded of how the subject can turn formerly peaceful liaisons momentarily sour. My in laws in the past once described me, or at least certain of those in the profession of which I am included, as being nothing more than 'charlatans', which may even be the correct perception. (The term 'charlatan' sounded more astounding when used in the Germanic intonation.)

Perhaps it is in part for these reasons I have attempted to make Trousers more about linking Design to something much broader, and not to be about linking anything to healthcare. As a result this stuff here on healthcare has been tucked out of the way and somewhat hidden at the end so as not to distract from the more important theme, being that of Design, as well as to be respectful of all the potential readers of this work, many sharing different opinion and experiences to my own.

I am not too sure how this discussion on healthcare will come across to someone who has not yet applied their senses toward understanding how they are influenced by their trousers, clothing, bedding, household articles and food. It could possibly be this all sounds too bizarre for contemplation, in which case or if that is a risk please focus on the information already provided and avoid considering the healthcare agenda until later. Making an active consideration of the senses and responses for healthcare is not a priority during the early stages of getting used to working with the responses as it is all quite an open ended discussion, without clarity, and so it could be potentially unhelpful, unsettling to a fledging in learning how to apply the senses and responses. Thinking about healthcare in this needs to be put out of one's mind when starting out in this, as it is more important to focus on developing one's ability to use the senses and responses for easier things whilst one learns how to work with them.

Therefore appendices 6 and 7 are specifically for those who are more inclined to think like myself, or as a result of having improved their ability to inhale with the diaphragm sufficiently to be able to response test with the aid of this alongside other observable responses to our world.

If you are continuing to read I am guessing you have worked out how to breath and can genuinely breath with just using the diaphragm. If so you may have also sorted out your trousers, and the rest of your wardrobe, according to your senses, improving your diet and your bedroom so these are also more response friendly. Alternatively, you may just be interested to consider healthcare before having worked with the senses, but please keep in mind how you perceive this all will change once you've been making use of the responses in ways suggested.

Whether or not it is achieved, or achievable, individuals should be better placed to make up their own minds on healthcare matters as a result of working with the senses and responses, as well as in determining their own personal strategy concerning keeping not just well, but in also finding something closer to the hallowed experience of 'perfect health'. However, regardless and in spite of our personal healthcare mantras, there will likely come a time for us all when we are faced with making quite serious choices regarding which of the health-care systems to go with, which of the two parallel systems and ways of thinking described in the part of this book about the X-system, even for something pretty minor like a mild infection, tonsillitis or a cold.

I have a regular patient who recently came down with a nasty cold, whilst staying out of the area, and she ended up going to the local doctor's surgery for help. The Doctor diagnosed tonsillitis and prescribed Penicillin and my patient phoned to ask me whether she should take it or not? (she was breast feeding and had concerns about her baby's milk supply becoming penicillin rich and uncertainty in how this might affect the baby).

Back during discussions on the X-system, and in consideration of the two parallel health management systems, I raised the idea that all is good as long as neither of these two systems interfered with the effectiveness of the other and I stand by this notion. However the problem runs deep when one comes to really contemplate the nature of each of these two parallel systems, just thinking about some of the themes covered in this book. Using the senses and responses is virtually akin to living off grid in 2013. In this current day you've got to be a bit of a devotee to the ideal to actually follow through with doing it.

I am not qualified or experienced to speak on our western, or the pharmacological, healthcare system, but am aware that often its approach cannot avoid compromising the X-system, and perhaps we have to just go with it in the same way we have been doing for a long time now. I am left asking myself whether any compromising of our X-system, possibly as a result of working with the more pharmacological and medical healthcare model, should really provide sufficient reason to avoid the multitude of benefits our pharmacological healthcare system is renowned at providing and we have become accustomed to receiving? Equally do we have to continue limiting ourselves, as we do, regarding our choices in healthcare, to this one system that tends to run us and takes the lead in organising and managing our provisions for healthcare to the more medical or pharmacological way of thinking? For myself I view the differences in the two healthcare systems as being not much different to those of being factory farmed, by way of the more pharmacological approach, as compared to my own seeking to be out there running free range and living organic, yet quite possibly also living in my own little fantasy world, engaged by way of the senses and responses. However as far as I can see both systems for our healthcare have their places in caring for us, yet at present how we work with health is one sided, at the expense of the system involving the senses and responses, and maybe it is now necessary to consider if or how we are loosing out as a consequence of this situation. Well, that is the position being put forward here in the hope of a consideration. I am putting these arguments forward in a way that is one sided, towards the idea of our better utilising the senses and responses, and be there no illusion that I am providing a balanced view, even though I am trying my best to do this.

In the past those the like of myself would have been branded as misguided and meddling loonies by the vast majority of those working within the pharmacological approach to healthcare. I need to add that the situation does not feel as though it has really much changed in recent years, simply because there is a lack of understanding over the sense based approach I have made attempt to describe. I think the matter as to whether I am misguided, or even a 'charlatan', can only be decided by those working within the pharmacological approach having a go at exercises to refine the use of the senses and responses as detailed. I do admit to meddling, and I must add there are many things to be said in the defence of the pharmacologically rooted system, based upon my own observations.

The thing is when we get ill, I see a part of the disease processes involves messing with our minds and the decision making processes. The end result leads us to easily ignore, or overlook, all the response based things we could do for helping ourselves, and immediately start to panic and look at our options in terms of the pharmacological healthcare system's view and way of thinking, because when we are ill we seem to automatically think more symptoms based as soon we are not at our best. This is something that can be tested when one is next sick or poorly with something, and is confirmed if we find ourselves grasping at a remedy for the symptoms rather than by way of an attempt at improving the senses and responses. A part of this phenomenon is in consequence of us being less able to trust our senses and responses when we are poorly, so it becomes more natural to seek our solution by thinking symptomatically. That's what the disease process does, and I'm under the belief that's perhaps how and why our society rolls as it does. And it's not the only thing that goes on with our brains when we are not at our best, which is something that becomes more and more apparent as a result of actually being able to engage the senses and responses in any decision making, including upon these matters about managing our own health and illnesses, and provides the basis for the broader picture I am aiming to connect with.

Onto practical matters. Consider a health remedy shopping trip to the health food store, or pharmacist, whether this is a virtual online store or located in a shopping centre. Think about how we have in the past been going about selecting our natural remedies for a specific problem or need we may have. How do we know whether what we are being recommended, either by the helpful staff or useful information on the label or other knowledge we have read or dug up on something, is really going to do anything for us, and will actually have the positive and noticeable impact upon what we are seeking remedy for? Then how do we know how much we should personally take of it to have this promised impact? If we are not being terribly careful all we are actually working with here is essentially just plain old fashioned faith medicine surely?

Then into the health food store or pharmacy, I have to say most are not response friendly in design and in fact many of these are very unfriendly for using the senses and responses. For myself, I would want to be able to go around testing things in my own way, just to gain an idea whether the advise being laundered my direction is potentially on track for me or not, by way of using my responses to go about double checking with. But here's a point, could it be these potentially less response friendly shops and purchasing means, that are so commonly used by us today for buying natural remedies, or buying anything else for that matter, actually sell more because we the consumer is either too uneducated about the responses, or just unable to apply the senses in those particular retailing environments, to make the more sense and response friendly purchase? The end result is possibly that we just end up buying more stuff than we potentially need in the hope of getting at least something right, like placing more bets to increase the chances that at least one of them might work out positive, a scatter shot approach to take them all in the hope we will hit the mark, completing this approach with a good measure of our old fashioned faith medicine, just in case the combination of it all does nothing for us.

Working more with the senses and responses is actually offering, as fringe benefit, the means of limiting what we consume, creating a more targeted approach for managing illness and maintaining health, but again please remember this is not all about health. Health itself has to be viewed as a fringe benefit in this, otherwise the health issue risks distracting the focus here.

How the health food and natural remedies industry has been in the past is not how it will be continuing, partially due to existing market forces. Yet if the consumer picks up on and starts using the senses and responses, in making purchasing decision, the way of things could get a whole lot different, even to the point of challenging those things currently forcing the market. We are taking about a complete revolution in thought and reason behind making purchases. What we are being sold may no longer remain what, from who or how we wish to buy our remedies in the future, at least for anyone utilising the senses and responses. Again this could apply to many if not all the things we purchase.

However, if we choose to generally make more response based decisions, we ultimately cannot avoid changing how we make our healthcare decisions. I provide another scenario to consider, we go find and visit the top natural healthcare practitioner or doctor we can, they are the Big Cheese, having plenty of qualification, reputation and standing. They give us nutritional advice on what we should and should not eat, along with providing us the remedies they recommend, and it is expensive, but we go with it as they have come highly commended and we haven't been recently feeling so good. When we get home what do we do? Do we follow their advice without question, do we just take what we are given and follow our instruction? I mean they are the expert, not us, who are we to question their authority? Let us not forget it was expensive the whole thing, the remedies we paid for and advice, what a waste if we don't comply? I have to add in the question, 'how many of our experts themselves engage in response testing or are openly encouraging of it?' Maybe they don't need to and are genuinely as good as their reputation.

Another scenario I encounter is holding off applying our own approaches to therapy, until the experts have given us the nod that this is all right for us to try out, and not trying out what our responses may be informing us of. Where in practice do we draw the line to define the extent that we, that's us, or our appropriately qualified specialist is appointed as the primary person in control of our care. This is if we are to consider there exist two parallel healthcare systems in operation, one of which we could potentially access, observe and manage, to some degree for ourselves.

We want to believe what we are informed about, as read on labels or in books, or of course on the Internet, or TV, about our natural and alternative remedies, like there is hope beyond the conventional way of things, and it is all interesting, it is indeed fascinating. But really, we have to ask how much of it does actually work for us as an individual, or is then the appropriate time to take it, and how do we recognise it is working? I say this because often we don't know and take things on good faith that they will be effective. Who should we believe, the experts or our senses and responses in this? Maybe there are some hidden pharmacological benefits our senses are unaware of, or maybe not? I do mean this really and am not being cynical. Over the years we have all heard so much authoritatively presented recommendation, much of it contradictory, from garlic is good for us, or is it now bad for us, or do this but not that, or that but not this. Come on, how do we know we fit the pattern of response these statements are based upon?

Personally I would not strictly follow what someone else says without double checking it for myself, but that's me. Too many people have vested interests in the business of health care, for ego and financial reason, or just deluded self faith.

Well that's how one has to be in business isn't it, make a sale by whatever means possible and hope that the customer is dumb enough to come back again? Now I am being cynical. There are also a great many good recommendations that may possibly work for us, provided by way of good reason and deduction, but should we still need to response double check the more trusted recommendations first, before popping whatever into our mouths or life? The system we have is really no different to gambling, where the odds are set against us, and sometimes we will get a win.

By the way, I do not trust my own advice without double checking it for myself. I think the primary aim concerning healthcare should be for the individual concerned to determine which of the systems any particular recommendation or therapy comes from, then at least we know from where they are working and how we are being treated. More things than we imagine are actually working with the X-sensory response system, it is just we have not been aware that this is how they are working in providing their acknowledged benefits. So the message is we need to get to know for ourselves which of our parallel systems the therapy is working through and we can do this by testing our responses before and after the therapy, it is as simple as that. As a result we should be able work out for ourselves what is really working best for us and then be in a position to lend useful feedback or make better decision regarding our therapies.

In the UK at the present time it appears that attempt is being made for the sense and response based system to be absorbed into the pharmacological system, or at least being invited to operate within the framework of our western pharmacological system, so that it can be promoted within the established State healthcare system, which sounds a fair enough proposal. So the question is, would it be an advantage to acknowledge the existence of two healthcare systems? Both systems are benefit providing, but differentiating them are the senses and responses. However within only one of these systems is it possible to sense our responses to the remedy or therapy. This defines the other system as being based upon pharmacology, chemistry, or direct physical intervention of the symptoms, which we cannot sense our responses to, yet it still helps us out.

Or, am I wrong here and there is in reality just one principle system, that which can be sensed by our responses, and anything that cannot be sensed as providing a positive response just does not work, and is in reality not what it is made out to be? This is not a statement but a question open for debate, to which I do not

Shaun M Sutton

know the extent of the answer because I mostly concern myself with the sense based system, and I do not wish to sound too ridiculous and to remain respectful of all the pharmacologically orientated therapies, utilsed to manage our hormonal and other bodily systems, and by which life is preserved.

Yet, could it be that in practice we are actually able to sense and response test all, or at least a greater proportion of our remedies, including those medicines of the pharmacological system and approach? Could it be that if the senses and responses reject it then it does not work at all, or that certain pharmacologically based remedies may just appear to work by way of unsettling the body's system to the point where it is doing something else, which ends up being incorrectly perceived as providing a benefit, when they are indeed far from genuinely useful?

Hopefully these questions may contribute to stimulating discussion, to be taken in the spirit of an open consideration upon matters that could only become clearer if and when mankind has evolved further in using the senses and re-sponses. Until then there is no clear way of learning what is the case, well at least not from me. Are these baffling and scientifically challenging questions, or just silliness on my part to debate? Although if we do not ask we just end up assum-ing something is the case, which may or may not be incorrect.

This is possibly not such a great place to end at in this work, yet it is in a way where I began. It is all a bit uncertain when all I personally cherish for in the world is more certainty to work with, and unfortunately I've added a lot of ques-tions without allowing for the practical aspects of managing such a complex mat-ter as healthcare. Added to my own world of uncertainty is the fact that our exist-ing primary healthcare system supports and inadvertently feeds the mindset that maintains the system, and billions of people rely upon this system, so I feel not much different to King Canute on the seashore shouting at the tide to go back when it is coming in. But this is not a work about healthcare, so I can hopefully excuse myself for any comments that cause offence, if that becomes necessary, and seperate myself from the subject, as I try my best to continue in doing.

One thing for me to make clear on, is that personally I have found it easy to become unduly embroiled in medical considerations as well as the politics of healthcare, and this takes up the mind, the thoughts, drives one further from the neutral place necessary to observe the senses and responses. When the mind becomes stuck into an analysis of such issues it is easy to overlook the other benefits from beyond the more medical way of thought, by way of applying the senses and responses. Thinking more symptomatically and analytically could, to some extent, be viewed as a trap that one has to pull oneself out from being drawn into, at least where working with the senses and responses are concerned. In some ways these two parallel systems cannot help being in conflict and naturally at odds with each other.

However all the time we each relinquish the control of what our senses and responses may to inform us of, to an authority beyond ourselves, there continues to exist an impass in the way of man's evolution towards something more than what we might now be achieving. Until the primary person in charge of our senses and responses becomes us, then any question in this regard remains unanswerable, so in a way the X-system may actually just remain my fantasy survival system of an elaborate imagination.

Maybe these are all matters which simply need to be ignored, just let the old world remain the old world, move on from its complexities and do our own thing to create the new world we individually desire for to happen, saving our breath, time and energy for what we can make easier influence upon for ourselves?

Appendix 7

Notes on using the senses and responses therapeutically

(continuing on from appendices 2 and 5)

To more fully appreciate the implications of therapeutically working with the senses and responses, it is probably ideal to have read appendix 6 before reading any further in appendix 7.

To perform a test of the responses to something it is simply a case of touching or holding it, or just letting it rest anywhere on the body. Measurement generally seems to be well perceived through materials like the fabrics of clothing, glass, plastic, paper, cardboard and pottery, so the article or material tested does not actually need to be directly touching the skin. (The other side to this phenomenon is that if you are carrying something compromising to your responses, this can potentially influence the X-system through these types of material)

These notes are provided as an extension on from appendices 2 and 5, and so need to be read with their context in mind.

If the diaphragmic inhalation count time, DICT (also referred to as LAPD within this book) decreases as a result of testing something, it should correspond with changes in the pulse such as a hardening, rising or pushing up of the pulse when tested, and indicates that just now this something can be considered as toxic to, or compromising of, the X-system.

If the DICT increases as a result of testing something, it should correspond with changes in the pulse such as an easing, relaxing, deepening, quietening and smoothing of the pulse, and indicates that just now this something can to be considered as therapeutic and benefiting to the X-system.

These examples of what can happen to the pulse when response testing are just several possibilities. In reality it is necessary to learn to observe how the pulse changes with corresponding changes in the DICT to get a feel for how these changes in the pulse actually feel to the individual.

If the pulse does not change with a corresponding change in the DICT then the change is being forced by way of the mind forcing the inhalation and therefore is most likely only an imagined change upon double checking. If you have found other aspects of the X-system you can objectively work with, they too would demonstrate a corresponding change in line with changes in the DICT and pulse.

The greater the increase or decrease of the DICT, when testing something, the greater that something's potential for therapeutic benefit, or toxicity and compromise, to the X-system.

Feelings are a potentially misleading subjective response and can prove to be especially misguiding for a novice at making decision based upon their senses and responses. Taking decision based on a feelings response alone has to be considered as an advanced means to work, and sole reliance on these could lead to errors in judgement for the novice. However it can be learnt to understand and trust the feelings more over time through observing how these alter in line with the other more objective (physically perceived) responses, allowing them to be introduced in a supportive role when working with the more objective responses. I still consider myself as a novice but do try to make my observations of subjective change for the sake of interest. My reliance on the more objective responses may be because I have had frequent times when my control over what I am thinking or feeling is poor.

It need be remembered with therapeutic items, which may be more traditionally considered as medicines (or therapeutic approaches), that what works today may only remain therapeutically active for a short while and then the body has changed and it works no longer, or alternatively the remedy may work for a period of days or even weeks before it no longer provides a regular beneficial response. However after then it could prove therapeutic again on some future occasion for that person, or maybe not, or need to be varied in some fashion. It can also be that something previously appearing as compromising to the X-system can, at a later date, become therapeutic. These comments on therapeutic things are based mostly on my own experiences in working with herbal medicines.

If someone suggests or gives you something to take, or you think you have found something by way of your own means to take for therapeutic effect, yet on testing it the pulse becomes harder, less relaxed and appears compromised, and the inhalation capacity lessened in the test, then what you have obtained will potentially have that exact effect of making the pulse harder, compromised and lessen the ability to inhale if taken internally. When something compromising is internally administered this effect becomes difficult to reverse, depending on how much has been administered and its potential degree of compromise. It is like being poisoned, although the effect is not fatal or strongly causing injury, but just be a bit inconvenient and unsettling to the senses and responses for a short while.

Alternatively, you have found or been given something to take for a specific reason, and your own response tests and other information you have to source cannot help in deciding whether you should or should not take it. Then the X-sensory response system will likely not be improved through taking it, in fact this something may in all likelihod compromise the system to some extent, especially if strongly therapeutic. I have often compromised my system, under similar circumstance, where I have relied upon 'hoping for the best' from something.

What do you do if you've compromised the system with something? If you cannot then find the remedy you then respond well to, being the antidote, perhaps even what you should have taken in the first place, then you've just got to get on in spite of, and ride it out the best you can for maybe an hour or two. If it's not poisonous and you take a remedy and it's incorrect for you, you could feel odd, or end up pacing about the house in the middle of the night, or turning over and over in bed cursing something or someone, quite possibly me, or just want to sleep during the day, or get a tummy ache, so it's no big deal really and is a part of the learning process if it happens. Some people are more robust than others to this, but the more potentially therapeutic the remedy, then the greater the risk of compromise to the system from the mistakenly taken remedy, although this is probably not entirely so. This is forgetting actual poisonous things, which are not being referred to here. (I did hear someone say that taking a hot bath could be a way of reducing the degree of such unsettlement by a non-poisonous remedy)

It is for these reasons why I don't personally take anything herbal or natural therapeutically if it shows no improvement in the responses on testing, regardless of the fact that it may be herbal and natural, or even organic or biodynamic. This approach saves my cash and time, and a lot of potential messing about if it all goes horribly wrong for me, even when I'm completely drawn to take something by way of mental deduction.

However there are those occasions when something appears to be testing well, but you aren't 100% sure on whether you are reading the responses correctly to be sure enough to take it, as you might be a bit stressed, rushed, tired or even ill. In these situations you can take the lowest safe dose you consider possible for the body to recognise whether it wants it or not, taking something like one 10th or 20th of the likely therapeutic dose, or even just a tiny taste, insufficient to unsettle the system if it turns out not to be something for you. Sometimes being apprehensive about taking something is for good reason, and there is no harm in being careful, in fact its quite a healthy sign. After taking this very small amount, and then re-testing, the response will hopefully have become more distinguishable one way or the other, but even then if there is a still a positive response do not necessarily just go ahead and take the full dose you think you could.

If you've not taken the remedy before, this is now beginning the process of identifying your optimum therapeutic dose, being the lowest dose at which anything further taken does not contribute to further beneficial changes in the responses.

It is something along the lines of the law on diminishing returns, where adding more, beyond a certain point, provides no further return, and maybe less return occurs from more. This is the point at which the optimum level of therapeutic change has already occurred for that specific remedy, and when re-checking the remedy, by touching it or its container, then no further response will be clearly recognisable. This may in some ways be likened to the workings of a canal lock. Once the water has filled it or been drained to be equal to that at the other side of the gate needing to be opened, that is the dose of water necessary for the lock to be opened, it is a set amount. In the case of the lock once the gates are opened everything can then flow through. It's not a perfect or completely accurate analogy, but it holds an interesting sentiment possibly helpful in understanding working therapeutically with the X-system.

So whilst there is a recognisable response when testing the remedy, and continuing to maintain the calm and impassive neutral mind, then more of the remedy can be taken, maybe beginning by just taking about a fifth to a tenth of the recommended dose at a time, and continue with retesting after each time of taking more, until the optimum therapeutic dose has been identified for that remedy, being when there is no more clear change in the responses when retested. I now work more cautiously with the responses because I have caught myself out on too many occasions and foolishly gone ahead and taken immediately the full dose of the remedy, I had thought was testing well. However it is only after, when I'm feeling a little odd, that I will reflect on how I had been a bit impetuous at the time and my mind had guided me in the decision more than my responses.

The mind's job in testing is to decipher what the senses and responses are informing it of and to work out how to act on the information being percceived. Its function in making decision is not that of making the selection for us without fully taking into account information provided by the senses and responses.

Even great masters, with the experience of practice make errors, and after many years of experience, but if they are working with therapies and remedies that will not kill you, then there is no real harm done, just no improvement and no benefit from the experience. This has been the traditional way of things with traditional medicine to a certain extent. A colleague told me of a valuable piece of experience given to them by a highly respected Japanese acupuncturist and teacher, the late Yanagishita Toshio Sensei, who was in practise for 62 years. Mr Yanagishita had indicated to them that he always tried to remain humble when treating and

Shaun M Sutton

allow for the possibility that he may have made an incorrect therapeutic decision or action causing a failed treatment, so he always tried to not be too certain about whether what he was doing would work in the way he hoped. It is important to allow for the possibility that what we think to be the case in testing things is actually not so. This helps ensure we are careful in what we are doing as a consequence of our testing with the responses.

Hopefully it is obvious to not go about testing and taking potential poisons or known poisonous substances this way, as it might be one fools oneself to believe it is acceptable and then it's too late afterwards, although it is interesting to test but not to take anything, and to see what we think about it with the responses. Caution is the word, move cautiously in these matters, be patient and take one's time. Never rush decisions in these matters under any circumstance, rushing a test is the time when the errors occur, being commonly when I have made many of mine. Work in the way that you feel comfortable with, and don't try taking self selected medicines this way until you feel you have learnt to trust your responses, then your body will also have become more resistant to the effects of getting it wrong, as eventually making errors in working with the responses are somewhat inevitable for anybody. I think that's how it goes. Remember there is not so much to gain by testing medicines this way until other things in your life have been changed to be friendlier to the senses and responses. Until other things have been made more response friendly there remains a lower margin for making errors in judgement of the responses. I make this point so that it is understood for your own safety. When you make errors in judgement with those other things in life that you may be testing these will not likely cause any harm, just the inconvenience of wasted time and error in your purchases or actions. However if it is a case of double checking a prescription you have been given, selected for you by a professional, then it should prove to be fairly safe and more straightforward to decide whether it is good for you or not when testing it with your own responses.

So in confirmation, if you wish to take something you consider the senses and responses are demonstrating improvement with, the correct dose is the dose taken at the exact point where no further improvement is being demonstrated by the senses and responses when testing and touching it, as compared to when not touching it. I find this generally becomes what I think of as a common therapeutic dose for that remedy, being the exact dose you can take again at a later stage to have the same effect whilst one remains responsive to that remedy. I have experienced a few occasions, with certain remedies, where at a much later date it is a significantly smaller measure that ended up as the optimum therapeutic dose, so caution is required. Sometimes at that later date the dose needed had increased also, so if you have not taken something for a while it is recommended to again do the step by step dosing, and re-testing at each step, with each further measure taken, until the optimum therapeutic dose is again reached. Generally though I have found that during any single period of time, for a remedy beneficial to the senses and responses, the optimum therapeutic dose will remain fairly consistently the same. My finding is that if you took that amount yesterday and it is showing a favourable response today, then the same dose will be sufficient each time you take it for the next few days or weeks, but still check if a lower dose works first before assuming, as the first time you may have been over dosing. This common therapeutic dose generally applies for another person, allowing something for an individual's weight, but you need to follow the senses and responses always, any theory in this is just helpful to begin, never assume theory is correct, especially one's own.

Occasionally it could be found, and especially when having a cold or a fever and treating oneself for it, the responses guide you to a remedy, you take it, find the optimum therapeutic dose and feel better, then 30-60 minutes later you feel the illness is returning, and the remedy still provides appearance of a beneficial response. Then just taking a half dose, half of what you just earlier took, has a good chance of being sufficient to be the required dose to clear and now knock whatever illness is bothering you on the head, at least for few hours with any luck. Be mindful of repeatedly dosing yourself this way with your common therapeutic dose, as during the delirium of being ill, or out of sorts, overdose is a high risk and to be avoided. You could be overdosing on something that is not what you are really needing just then to improve the responses, and this could also be why the responses are not holding for that long after taking your remedy. It is all too easy to make errors, especially when ill or feverish, so being aware of this can help reduce the occurrence of errors by more closely careful obsevation of the responses.

I have sometimes found that the recommended dose on a packet is quite insufficient to have the optimal therapeutic effect, and is significantly less than what I have found to be this common therapeutic dose, so taking something at the suggested dose can do very little, even if the responses indicate it helps. Often I find it necessary to take quite a bit more, but this does depend on the source for the dosage information, so there are no hard rules, other than caution, as often the dose suggestions are also quite accurate.

The point to stop taking further measures of something is the point where you are unsure if the responses, from testing something, through holding or touching it, are any better as compared to when not testing it, allowing for the risk of over enthusiasm unsettling the senses and forcing a false positive from their reading. I have often been just at that point spooning another measure into my mouth and stopped myself, retested, and find I've already had enough, and have in fact taken what is the optimum therapeutic dose for that remedy for me at that time.

When seeking to find the optimum therapeutic dose for a remedy, with each further measure taken the difference in the responses between when touching the remedy and when not touching it will lessen each time, until the point of there being no difference. When there is no more response no more remedy is taken.

In terms of regularity of dose, this varies from remedy to remedy and condition to condition. Normally three or maybe four times a day is the maximum frequency for use of a remedy, but during a cold or fever illness this frequency could be traditionally increased upon, with caution and definitive guidance coming from the responses. There are many occasions when taking something just once or twice a day is all the responses are indicating as appropriate, sometimes even once every other day, so there are no rules other than to follow the responses and be mindful to not overdose due to enthusiasm or being overly neurotic. I think the ideal is to make time to test possible remedies 3 to 4 times a day, at regular intervals, to see what you think of the responses for yourself, and then take it whenever the responses indicate a definitive benefit is being demonstrated. This is opposed to only taking something once a day because of the inconvenience to test more often. To some extent this matter of frequency becomes a personal choice, and if you are just drawn to test something when you remember maybe that is the best way to be working with remedies and the responses. I am being serious, as it allows one to get on with life, but I test remedies 3 to 4 times a day.

I have heard of reliable professionals recommending people to take a lower starting dose in case of healing crisis, in order to lessen the degree by which symptoms can occasionally become worse whilst the body is actually improving and correcting itself, which could support the idea of taking a remedy less regularly than is recommended. By taking a lower than recommended dose the changes are more gradual and so any symptomatic worsening, associated with improvemment, remains milder, and people are not put off taking the medicine or made anxious because of conditions worsening, where associated with what could be considered a healing crisis. I'm not sure about how or if this matter of the symptoms getting worse before they improve happens when working with feedback for frequency and dose being provided by the senses and responses, as it may be the body somehow recognises this healing crisis issue and the feedback automatically reduces the dose taken based on the response testing. However it is best to assume healing crisis may still occur, at least in the beginning of taking natural remedies, plus there may also be errors in one's judgement of the responses, especially for the novice, so always taking perhaps a little on the less side, than the more side, is the recommendation, helping to reduce the risks of error.

In herbal therapy there commonly exists the professional recommendation to continue taking a remedy for a while longer than the moment more chronic or longer term symptoms have cleared up, the intention in this being to reduce the chance of these symptoms reoccurring. It may be a similar observation is made when working under the guidance of the senses and responses, where principal symptoms clear up yet the responses still indicate continuing on with that remedy. When using the senses and responses as guide the symptoms are in a way just to be viewed as another of the responses, being observed and taken into account alongside all other responses, that is as opposed to the symptoms constituting the only response being noted. I tend to notice that if I have been taking a remedy for more than just a few days, and the responses have been initially very favourable and clearly readable, there comes a time where the benefit observable when testing, or as a result of taking that remedy, is no longer so dramatic or clear. I take this as an indication that the usefulness of the remedy is coming to an end. However in this situation a complete change does not tend to happen all of a sudden with the responses indicating "That's enough, job done, thank you very much", as there could be some number of days over which the responses test positively or the experience when taking the remedy is favourable, intermixed with days where I'm feeling there is no benefit going fromit. This time frame of mixed responses may help explain and confirm the recommendations made by professionals working differently to myself, when encouraging the longer use of a remedy or medicine. I tend to seek a replacement remedy on these occasion and even end up having a period of time taking a fresh remedy during one part of the day and the former at another time. Patterns of response often begin to show.

Extending on from this I have at times experienced an intermediate condition, observed as such as a result of my using the diaphragmic inhalation count time, the DICT, as one of the judges for my response to a remedy. This intermediate condition comes across as the count time dropping for the same remedy that had just a couple of days or so previously been providing a much higher count when testing, yet still the count when testing remains significantly higher than when not testing the remedy. This has often culminated with me finding it possible to adapt the remedy's recipe (combination of therapeutic ingredients) in someway, where certain of the components are deemed by the senses and responses as no longer required or other things may now be included. Certainly this is a technical matter more for the clinician, but because of its practical significance this could prove useful for the patient to keep in mind. Anyone who has been working upon developing the DICT response would be better placed to make use of this information, as differences observed from testing become more perceivable when working with the DICT as a gauge of response. The end result would be that if the formulation of the remedy can be adjusted, to provide an increase in the DICT, there would also be an improvement in the other responses being observed. My feeling is that by working in this way, to increase the DICT, allows for a greater opportunity of observing certain problematic symptoms as resolving or lessening in their severity, in line with higher levels observed for the DICT.

I need remind the reader, and myself, that I am just speaking here about my own experiences in using the responses therapeutically, and it is important to recognise these are merely based upon my own observations. I reflect that I may have ended up working this way because of something in my character or situation preventing me from working in the more usual and accepted ways, also being the time tested ways for many forms of traditional medicine. As observed during my participation in the Japanese Kampo herbal therapy, where the experience and skill of the herbal practitioners seemed to somehow naturally take into account the same things my own senses and responses were informing me of. There will surely be many ways of achieving the same end result, I think that is what I wanted to say. I mix my therapies when treating myself, finding each achieves something slightly different, but all have in common the same connection, the X-system, this is what unifies my differing approaches.

How I go about all this is just the way I personally evolved into, a way suiting me. How others work with the X-system maybe cannot help but be different, and yet still work for them, but is just in a style of approach suited to their own person and circumstance. Perhaps we can all be right in how we go about things, each means of approach having its strengths, making up for its weaknesses, each maybe more suited to some people and not others. Treating symptoms of disease through working with the senses and responses for me is a vague and non-exact matter, so I hope these descriptions can help do some justice in support of this point, making for some clarity within the misty zone of therapeutic approaches and the senses and responses. It maybe I'm adding to the fog.

Out of all the remedies available, several of the simplest and most effective are to take a walk outside or to sit quietly reading an old fashioned paper book, a novel, or reading something that is not so meaningful and is un-stimulating on the mind in some way. From my own experience I have at times worked myself to be unsure or anxious upon what my responses are or are not informing me of, yet it has also ended up as being surprisingly easy to calm myself down again once I accepted this as being the case. Try to avoid working oneself up if you cannot clearly read the responses, or if they are making no sense, and certainly before any harm occurs though uneducated or reckless actions based on what you imagine they are indicating. Learn to recognise this situation should this be you. If this is something you have become aware may be a problem for you, learn when to stop testing with the responses and to give it a break, allowing the mind to fully regain more calm. Too much testing, added with a degree of anxiety because you cannot feel quite as right as you would like, can end up over stimulating the thoughts, so that needs to be arrested before re-testing anything further with the responses. It may be you are actually fine and there is nothing at all wrong, and it was literally all in the mind, like a panic attack or hysteria. I've suffered from both, the hysteria crept up on me and I had to learn to recognise it and ease back somehow by doing nothing, giving testing a break. This could commonly occur if I was hungry or thirsty, or missed out on our more obvious needs, including that of just becoming calm by whichever means were available and seem to best nurture my inner quiet.

When taking herbal formulas I tend to avoid taking more than two different formulas at any one moment. Taking just one is more ideal perhaps, less being best. Definitely avoid taking anything just for the sake of it, unless you are certain your responses will show an improvement as a result. I think there are too many health conscious people who are overly conscious and take as great or a greater number of things that are as compromising for them, as compared to those things demonstrating benefit, where the responses are concerned. Test what you want and take what appears to be working or not and you may notice what I mean. Just take one thing only at any one time to begin with, so you can work out what is or is not working out for yourself.

Where general health supplements are concerned, I guess you can think of them as foods, maybe they don't have a negative impact on the responses but are just neutral. You have to question your reasons for carrying on with taking anything that is neutral in response. Maybe a proper fresh meal might be a better option? I would question taking any supplement that tests out to be neutral and especially if compromising to the responses, so you have to ask yourself why take it? Ah as a kind of insurance policy, then I suppose that will be fine then, you need to decide from your own senses in this.

If you are recommended to take something by a professional and it does not test well, it may be it's effects are pharmacological, even if it is all natural, organic or herbal, and this is something I am not able to comment upon, especially if this is a prescription medication. My recommendation is to be sure you are actually gaining something from taking it, and that you remain understanding of its effects on your responses. It maybe the dose you take is insufficient to leave the responses worse off, or seriously compromised, so take the recommended dose and see, or try out a little and see. Don't make any decisions on what you think until you have actually taken it a few times whilst testing it with your responses, just in case you are suffering from a neurosis and you simply imagined it to compromise your responses, when maybe this was just a case of imagining the worse from it.

My contention is too many things just get taken without being questioned. Do not stop taking any medicines prescribed by a physician without consulting that physician first or getting a second opinion from a similarly qualified person. Always err on the side of caution in what you do or do not use, and always follow the instructions you are provided with, but don't give up your own right to seek counsel from your senses and responses if you have been training with them. It may seem intimidating to do, but question the professional prescribing the medicine to ask if it is really necessary for you to take it, if you happen to find it is repeatedly and significantly compromising your responses when tested and actually internally taken, and ask of your other options under their care? There is always the possibility the professionals you are working with actually appreciating your feedback, and candidness, in this as its also in their interest that you get well. And finally, ensure the packaging your medicine or remedy comes in is not compromising your responses. I for instance am unable to test anything in a metal or foil container because I do not respond well to that material. So don't be foiled by the packaging! It may be you response test a pharmaceutical medicine and believe it to compromise your responses, but in fact it is just the blister pack it is contained within causing the problem identified with the responses.

Keep in mind it is the X-system being worked with here, so there will be a multitude of responses occurring. If you are working with observing the pulse and breath, keep a look out for other things changing as a part of the X-system during tests or when taking something you are responding to. The greater the variety of responses you are able to observe and work with, the better the decisions you are able to make. Using both the pulse and breath together is a good way to double check on each, and to learn about how each correspondingly changes in response, so this idea can help in checking on and learning of other responses.

Another response to experiment with testing is how the pulse changes under each of the middle three fingers, independently of each other, which provides a more refined method of working, as you will notice the pulse under each can change differently with the responses. Just recently I experienced a few occasions when my pulse character changed from its usual regular pre-test picture, baffling me by becoming less forceful, and made the pulse more difficult for me to read and understand my responses by way of it. Then I had to become more aware of how the pulse changed in line with changes in the breath to find my remedy and observe what was then changing, especially taking notice of the pulse under the index finger's location, as the pulse was disappearing from there when not holding the remedy, and returning there again when holding the remedy. I tend to take most notice of what happens to the pulse under the index finger, but the other fingers help to support the findings, especially the middle finger.

In terms of the accuracy of decisions being made about which remedies to take, decisions have the greater possibility of inaccuracy when the selection is based upon purely theoretical analysis, unless that person has mastered working in this way and even then just working according to theory has it's risks of inaccuracy. The more accurate means of making selection is by applying two or more tests of the X-sensory response system, excluding any symptomatic complaint, which allows for the more immediately changing responses to be compared against each other, ensuring beneficial response is actually occurring, in addition to initial support guidance provided by theory or experience in the selection process.

Shaun M Sutton

Applying theory and experience to selection provides benefit in widening the choice of possible remedy, through a deeper knowledge of remedies, their therapeutic actions and guiding principles, whilst at the same time reducing the number of remedy or action options, by way of what is indicated in the theoretical information or from experience about the instances where that remedy or action does and does not particularly apply. If it is possible to double check on theoretically made decision, with the senses and responses, before theory's application, this helps confirm if the theory was being interpreted correctly, or even if the theory is actually correct or applies in this situation.

In another article I literally just happened upon whilst going through the back issues of my NAJOM journal, this time from November 1995, Miki Shima, OMD, L.Ac., and a former student of Tadashi Iriye the inventor of the Finger Test, wrote something close to this matter which also helps expand upon sentiments developed from my own observations.

"If one relies only on the intuitive aspect of the healing system, one is very prone to make mistakes. If one depends only on the rational differential diagnosis, one cannot utilise intuition, which is tremendously important."

As earlier indicated it is my opinion that one of the finest remedies to consider is to find some nature to hang out in for a good while, it is so simple it is all too easily overlooked. Sometimes when we are not well it is necessary to literally drag ourselves away from our somewhat pressing indoor activities, commitments or tasks, to get ourselves outdoors in order to eventually gain some better clarity in our perspective. Often, if we do a good job with contacting nature this way, after a while outside, we realise what we had previously thought to be so pressing isn't really that necessary after all. This may be testimony to the extent our relationship to the natural world has become derogated in our functional environments.

This all provides for a challenging maze to work through, so just start at the beginning, start at the trousers, get used to testing clothing first and improve one's living conditions, according to the responses, as the immediate priority. Working with the responses to medicines can be worked up to after these priority things have been first improved, so healthcare is really the last thing to consider in relation to the responses, in an ideal world. Or you can do it like me, just do it, make lots of errors, half poison yourself at times, all for the sake of trying one's best to live by way of guidance from the senses and responses, which maybe helped me more quickly learn how to use them, I'm not sure.

When considering the familial connections discussed in Part IX, this clearly broadens view on the impact of our individual material decisions upon those closest to us, linked together by our unseen energetic connections. On some level not everyone in the family needs to go so sense and response friendly, if we are able to look to ourselves for remedy and thereby influence others this way. Perhaps it found possible for the family unit to gain more if those we are intimately connected with are also involved with living respectfully of their sesnes and responses? However I am also thinking we need to be able to make our own choices, and matters of these kind cannot be demanded of or forced upon anyone, regardless of the potential benefits. Any ideas of enforcement doesn't feel right somehow. Yet, I still question the extent placing the priority upon satisfying the needs of one's own senses is able to accomadate issues with those we are intimately connected to, for instance if our intimates are practicing material and lifestyle choices compromising to ourselves by way of the same energetic connections.

As for identifying the 'perfect health' condition, through working with the senses and responses it is likely to become clear that perfect health can be viewed as an ever changing and momentary state. However there are to be found times when there is nothing further to be gained through therapeutic engagement of the X-system. This is where the body has pretty well righted itself as best as is possible at that time and cannot be righted further. When working with observing the diaphragmic breath, something closer to perfect health is experienced when the ease and capacity of diaphragmic inhalation is at its maximum. For myself a most important of responses I engage is that of how well I am sensing and interacting with my immediate environment, which seems to be associated with my not thinking about much of anything at that time. If I think, I sense less, and may play a part in why perfect health only ever seems to be momentary, at least to me. These experiences can reflection upon what may have influenced us in feeling well, even if momentary, and are helpful in learning about ourselves.

Recommended reading to compliment the medical discussion

East Asian Medicine in Urban Japan by Margaret M Lock, first published 1980, University of California Press

Feeling the clear

Lunchtime after rain showers
the air becomes still,
or at least now I feel the stillness.

Yellow shouts in my face
leaps across from distant autumn trees,
jumping up from the grass,
fallen leaves,

Each and every moment unique
continuation of the clear breath,
feels like rain drenched foliage
around an absent woodland pool.

Bird song from each direction
carried on breath's plane,
crystal clear their droplets,
notes falling from the sky.

Appendix 8 - design in practice using senses of response -

Recreating ancient therapeutic products

Concerning design, as a student and practitioner of East Asian Medicine, instead of working in the field of designing and manufacturing a meal, clothing, furniture, a room set, office space or a home, my business is in designing of a therapy in attempt to match the unique needs brought to me by each of my customers. However, where working with the senses of response are concerned, I am completely certain that a similar set of principles must exist between those needed in my designing of a therapy as compared to those, for instance, in designing a living or bedroom in a home. The difference between the two is that the requirements of the therapy may possibly be more single person specific, as compared to when designing anything else, or at least this is what I am thinking whilst taking into consideration these senses and responses within my own work. In reality working with senses and responses may turn out as being something of a single person specific matter.

The best thing I might possibly offer is describe what is involved for me in utilising the senses and responses, within design processes of my own work. My example is provided in describing how I go about refining a traditional herbal formula's recipe, in this case a combination of therapeutic materials originally described in an ancient Chinese text, from the initial matters I have to contend with, through to re-assembling the formula's recipe in such a way as to achieve some significant improvement in the starting formulation, as determined by observing the senses and responses. This hopefully should provide some insight into what goes on for me, and general idea on what could potentially be involved in designing anything, when ultimately considering benefit to the senses and responses of the user as a non-negotiable within design processes. When I mean anything, this literally is in designing and manufacturing anything humans intimately engage with.

There exist established ways in doing anything for best effect, and in herbal medicine these are really quite varied, as in doing anything else. How I work myself with herbal medicine is not a traditionally taught or the standard approach, as one, being what evolved as working for me. As indicated, in appendix 7, there can be considered many ways of seemingly achieving the same end therapeutic goal, as gauged by beneficially influencing the senses and responses.

The means by which I reproduce these traditional herbal formulas includes my referring to various books and notes assembled for my study, several of which are from the direct translations into English of more modern reproductions of ancient Chinese texts, from the Japanese or Chinese languages which I cannot read, written by various authors, detailing actual recipes for the different herbal formulas traditionally used as medicines in the East Asian culture, what it is each formula treats in the person, and clues about what to look for in a particular person to assist making a correct selection of any single formula, from the wide range of formula recipes available to me. From my view, the correct selection is that particular traditional therapeutic recipe I find as demonstrating the greatest improvement in the senses and responses of the person it is to be used by.

I find the observation striking how an English person, with no Asian parentage, living in England during the 21st century, can demonstrate positive responses to ancient Chinese herbal recipes, many originally recorded some 2000 years or more ago, and made up using fairly simple natural raw materials, most of which are not native to the English shores. As a consequence of my being a relative novice, in working with these ancient recipes of therapeutic repute, I have been regularly left unclear of what the information in any particular text may actually mean to me in practice, as a result of holes in my knowledge and inconsistency between the texts and notes at hand, about what each say about the same recipes. Some of such issues are likely responsible in encouraging my use of the senses and responses to navigate my way around this subject, being something I have been troubling over for a number of years.

Sometimes texts will indicate certain of the ingredient components need to be processed in some way or other, for instance by being cooked in wine, baking, or blending with honey, sometimes not, sometimes certain ingredients are always the processed version, and often the same ingredient may be processed in different ways to achieve what may appear to be the same end result. Then, at least in the more ancient reference texts, ingredients can be given in an ancient form of measure, that has to be translated to a modern measure, and I have come across various ideas upon what that actually translates to in modern measure, and sometimes several forms of measure are given within the same recipe, as volume and weight, whereas I only work by weight. The texts may also suggest possible ingredient additions or subtractions from a recipe, under certain special circumstance, that may not be completely clear for me to understand in practice. So my difficulty is that of different experts saying different things, or that certain things may have ended up being overlooked or lost during all the translation processes over the years.

A big issue, for perhaps all practitioners working with the more traditional of herbal formulas passed down through the ages, is that certain of the ingredients are currently banned or restricted in their use, for a variety of reason, or are just now unavailable, and so these certain ingredients may require equivalent substitution to be identified in fulfilling their role within a recipe. However there is little or no traditional practice existent to support using many of the suggested modern substitutions within these particular recipes. Equally, from the same texts, the overall majority of the formulas detailed can be made with what is readily available, and according to the recipes provided for each.

It is at this point I should try to make clear why I see one would work with therapeutic formulas, containing a number of individual materials within their recipe, other than this being to follow the teachings of a traditional practice. Essentially, from the view of working with the senses and responses, it is that the effect of two ingredients combined is greater than of just one, three than two, etc, etc, until a formula recipe is completed to suit treating the characteristics of the person it has been traditionally used to assist. I will refer to this use of multiple compounds, combined within any specific recipe, as a 'layering' of therapeutic compounds, achieving the greater effect from the recipe than from just using each material it contains singularly or fewer individual ingredients in combination than is the given for use in a particular recipe.

The next issue is, when working with Chinese medicines in our modern times, there exists opportunity to employ the use of a concentrated extract form for each potential ingredient, produced in dissolvable powder or granule form, so that it is no longer necessary to use the original form for each ingredient in the most common traditional way for the recipe's preparation, generally that of all being boiled up together in water for a while, sufficient to reduce the liquid down to about half the original volume, ensuring all that is necessary has been extracted from the ingredients in the recipe. Guidance is given on how much modern concentrate is equivalent to using the original raw version for each ingredient, but there exists a number of manufacturers producing these concentrates so a question remains over whether they are all equivalent in their concentration from the perspective of dose, in spite of each manufacturer's indications, and whether the recommendations on conversion between concentrated granules and the original raw form for materials are accurate.

I have also studied with expert practitioners who each consider things quite differently over the matter of whether anything necessary is lost from the original raw ingredient material, during the process of producing the modern concentrate, leading to a reduction in effectiveness for a formula's recipe. I have also come across instances where these same raw materials have been provided in the form of strong alcohol extracts and dispersions, but have not myself much used or experienced this more modern form for using these particular ingredients within the traditional formulas I am re-creating.

For reason of convenience, and experiment, I generally end up using certain of the ingredients in their original raw form, being dried roots, barks, fruits and seeds, in making up a formula's recipe. This is achieved by way of my earlier having ground each of these particular ingredients into a very fine powder, then used the powder I have made for an ingredient either to complete a recipe, when mostly using the ingredients in the modern concentrated extracted form, because the extract form for a particular ingredient required to complete a recipe is currently unavailable to me, or alternatively I will use the original raw herb form for majority of the different ingredients, ground into their powders, then adding the remaining ingredients in the modern concentrate form, because I am unable to successfully grind those from their original raw form into the fine powder I need for working in this way. Using the raw ingredients in this fine powdered form allows them to easily be mixed with the concentrated granules and the dosage for the recipe to be taken fairly conveniently, mostly through being added to a cup of boiling water. Working with my own powders of the original raw materials perhaps saves me some money, as the raw original herb is a bit cheaper to use although less convenient because of the need to grind it, plus I am interested to investigate whether the original, or its concentrated form, provides any better result when considered against the senses and responses.

Finally there is the consideration of whether we are certain the quality of the ingredients being used is not varying in some way, between different suppliers or batches, although my own herb suppliers do perform tests on what they receive to potentially help in managing this. However I am unsure as to whether the quality of what is available today is not different in some way to when the recipes I am working with were originally created, many being over 2000 years old.

As I am going to be using the senses and responses, with which to test the efficacy of these traditional herbal recipes, I first need to actually assemble each formula's recipe in order to initially go about my testing processes, making up some of the recipes according to my most trusted texts, whilst taking note of what other texts also say about the formula concerning traditional forms of processing certain components and what to look for in the person that the recipes are indicated for use with. Eventually I have built up a number of my 'best estimations' of different traditional Chinese herbal recipes.

When I am working to treat myself with these Chinese herbs, whilst the various responses I work with could be many, I always include making use of the DICT (an abbreviation for the 'diaphragmic inhalation count time' - see appendix 2 for more information) and pulse responses, especially when it is necessary to initially work out any refinements within the formulation of components in a recipe. In fact the only time I can actually refine my best estimation recipes, to be more beneficial upon the senses and responses, is when I or someone else is actually responsive to that particular recipe at that precise moment in time. I am then provided with the unique opportunity to more precisely work out that formula's recipe in practice, with guidance during the refinement process coming from observations of the senses and responses.

When someone is actually found to be responsive to one of the 'best estimation' formula recipes I have recreated, where I felt a discrepancy existed between texts on the use of either the processed or unprocessed form for a particular ingredient, now is the time for these different ingredient forms to be tested against the responses, so that the most effective upon the responses can be identified for further use in the recipe. If any ingredients are unavailable, and substitution is a possibility, now is also time to test these against the responses as well. 'Making hay when the sun is out' sort of thing. If my initial best recipe estimation, that has been selected to work with by the responses, then needs to be altered according to what has been learnt during these checks, this is carried out immediately and constitutes the making of a 'first stage in refinement' to the recipe. This may require a complete remaking of the recipe from scratch, if possible there and then, in the cases where I had not earlier utilised the best of ingredient forms from the view of the responses.

Shaun M Sutton

Once a potentially beneficial formula has been identified, and any first stage in refinement is completed, it is necessary to then double check any first stage refinements prove themselves to actually be correct, by way of applying the processes described in appendix 7, identifying the optimum therapeutic dose for a remedy. Once this has been completed, and the newer re-creation of the recipe proves to generate a greater beneficial response, than that for the earlier best estimation, then a 'second stage in refinement' to the recipe becomes possible.

The second stage in refinement is to identify which of the component materials, in the recipe being worked with, continues on in providing some level of benefit, as observed by the senses the responses, after the optimum therapeutic dose for the stage one refined recipe has been measured in. When the body has had enough of something the responses are indicative of this, and whilst certain of the components in a recipe may individually continue to demonstrate some further possibility of beneficial response, to other of the components the responses will indicate that enough has been already been measured in. It had appeared to me that these response spent components are what now restricted further beneficial response from being observed, even though other components continue on in demonstrating this response is possible for them. I imagine this is some sort of basic law, similar to something I cannot recall the name for, concerning a bottle neck generated by what I now consider to be a greater need, than is being satisfied, for certain components within the formula's recipe. This means, for the purposes of the second stage in refinement to a formula's recipe, the aim is to identify which of the component ingredients continue to exert a beneficial response, by way of their insufficiency, within the formulation of recipe.

When working out a recipe I often make the second stage in refinement at some later time, after the first stage has been completed, due to insufficient time and a risk of over exerting use of the senses and responses. However if I remain fresh for the purpose in hand I carry straight on into the second stage directly, after the first stage is completed, taking opportunity in the moment. However, when treating a patient I commonly stick with the first stage refined recipe or even just the best estimation I originally made up, at least for a while, going on to investigate the further stage in refinement to a recipe if it continues to demonstrate the same positive responses over time. Working without rushing the refinement process helps in being certain about the appropriateness of a refinement, as well as in lessening the risks associated with overworking the senses and responses, being emotional and response unsettlement, leading to error of judgment.

To begin the second stage in the refinement process for a recipe, a fresh starting point for the responses first needs to be clearly established and noted before any further refinement can be assessed by the responses. This is a case of assessing how much the body organism has just beneficially altered, directly after and as a result of having taken the optimum therapeutic dose of the first stage refined recipe, from both an objective perspective as well as any possible subjective means recognised to successfully gauge a potential for refinement. Once the level or degree of existent response to a recipe has been assessed, and gauged by the responses, each component in the recipe is then individually introduced to the body, by way of holding, touching or placing the component, or the container holding it, on the body in the usual manner when response testing.

If it is possible to work with the DICT response this could prove especially helpful as a gauge of response with which to work, although so far I have only managed to use the DICT when working just with myself, although my patients are commonly good at indicating their subjective observation to help confirm and support what I may be observing objectively in their responses. However I find it helpful to appreciate that whatever was the level of the DICT, when testing a component ingredient, will be the same level attained after that component's optimum therapeutic dose has been taken, with similar observation also being the case for all other responses observed and worked with. If making consideration to the subjective response, components continuing to demonstrate a beneficial response seem to provide for an immediate sense of relaxation or uplift, a calmer mind or clearer appreciation of the senses to ones immediate environment, but the degree of this often seems to be greater when actually taking it, as opposed to when the component is just being response tested.

Any components demonstrating a response further on from what had already been achieved, from that of a short while earlier when the first stage refined recipe was taken, are then individually taken according to the process, described in appendix 7, for finding the optimum therapeutic dose for a therapeutic remedy. Any further amounts taken, for the recipe's individual components, are carefully measured and noted, during this process of the second stage in refinement, until each provides no further beneficial response when re-tested.

The 'first stage refined' recipe can now be adjusted according to any extra amounts taken for the component parts. This is probably simpler math than may appear to be the case. If, for instance, around 28% of the quantity originally made of the first stage in refinement recipe produces the optimum therapeutic dose response, then this would require making an addition of amount to a component in the recipe taken during the second stage to the quantity of

100/28 multiplied by the extra amount of that component taken during the second stage in refinement.

What I find more complicated is the math to bring the remainder of the first stage in refinement recipe up to the equivalent of those proportions now indicated for the ingredients, as a result of the second stage in refinement additions for components. To ensure error in the math does not occur I write down all my calculations, so these can be reviewed again if I want to double check the math, as it would be a shame for mathematical mistake to be a cause for error after all this work. Then the amount taken to produce the optimum therapeutic dose for the first stage refined recipe needs to be increased accordingly, from a theoretical view, to allow for any extra taken for individual components, although this may be best double checked with the senses and responses in case somehow the second stage in refinement recipe requires a different dose than imagined theoretically. However I have tended to find that the theoretically increased dose for the recipe to be the correct one. Therefore in this case the proportion of the optimum therapeutic dose would still be 28% of the total amount in the recipe, as long as quantities remain as per the original first stage in refinement recipe, plus any amount added as consequence of the second stage in refinement.

For some of my earlier refined formula recipes I have re-done the second stage refinement at a much later date, checking and refining further if needed. This is especially appropriate if I reflect as to having introduced some level of theory into the earlier refinement in deciding the amount for a particular component to be used. Again the formula always needs to be providing a continued beneficial response with which to refine from.

Working in the way I do enables me to immediately test which of my texts and translations, covering the use of these traditional therapeutic formulas, are most accurate, by agreeing with my own findings upon the processing form used for ingredients, the individual levels of component proportion and overall recipe dosage. As such these texts then become my more valued in helping to make up my initial best estimations for future formula recipes I re-create, and so hopefully I can go on to observe better and clearer response before any refinements are necessarily undertaken than would otherwise have been the case. As for which texts are most agreeing with my own refinements, I have not found one which is perfect in its recommendations, so considering a number of them still remains my most beneficial proposition, although my response observations have tended to find greater agreement with the most ancient recordings upon the formulation of these traditional therapeutic recipes.

Whilst there may still exist the possibility to further modify a traditional formula's recipe, beyond the second stage in refinement, by way of an appreciation for some potential new ingredient addition to further benefit the responses, this is perhaps best tested for on another occasion, unless the work to this point has been particularly easy and straightforward, again because of the risks associated with over testing during one sitting. It could be better to try out what has been refined first for a while to ensure it demonstrates consistent and repeated benefit for the responses, again something that is only possible whilst the recipe remains appropriate for the person being worked with. Often I am unbelievably tempted to try some further new addition to the recipe's formulation immediately, after the second stage in refinement, out of curiosity, but what was it they said about curiosity and the cat? I therefore follow the guidance of certain acupuncture teachers who suggest enough has been done during a treatment session when you begin questioning whether enough has been done.

When the recipe has been built and adjusted, according to the second stage in refinement, if the DICT can be measured along with other responses, it should become clear that this particular formulation for the recipe repeatedly improves the DICT to the same point of response each and every time the optimum therapeutic dose is taken, as long as all other variables remain the same for that person. This would be a quite specific DICT, (in my case it could be a DICT of something like 35), and be around double the level of my DICT response before anything is taken (in my case generally the starting level for my DICT response is around 15-20). However, I am aware that a really great therapeutic recipe, for benefiting my own responses, will generate a DICT to the level of at least two and half to three times the starting level of response (so in my case this can be a DICT of at least 45 and commonly more than 50), upon taking the optimum therapeutic dose. Therefore if the DICT response level for myself were just double the starting level of response, after the optimum therapeutic dose for a second stage refined recipe is taken, I am aware something new could potentially be added to improve the responses further towards my highest level of response.

Shaun M Sutton

This is investigated within of a 'third stage in refinement' to the recipe's formulation, through 'modifications and additions', testing out new potential component ingredients.

Modifications and additions to a particular recipe's formulation are commonly indicated in reference texts. A modification to the classical version of an oriental herbal recipe's formulation can be by the way it is presented for use, such as mixed up with honey, alcohol or with rice gruel, or by way of the addition of other traditional medicinal materials to the refined recipe, as an additional individual herbal component, combination or another complete traditional recipe formulation. The modification or addition is appropriate if the responses indicate a benefit when testing the new ingredients prior to or after the optimum therapeutic dose for the refined formulation has actually been taken. I have tended to try it both ways on different days to be sure the modification is genuinely working with the refined recipe's formulation and not having any adverse influence on the responses, possible as a result of an earlier misgauged modification or addition decision.

However when carrying out the third stage in refinement to a recipe generating beneficial response, by way of modification or addition, I generally test and then take any potential modifying or additional components before taking anything of the second stage refined formula because I find it quicker and easier to assess the responses then (If there is confusion over how this is achieved, I have to test the recipe first, so as to ascertain the recipe remains or is appropriate, using the means described in appendix 7, then hold off taking it until after the addition or modification is worked with). If an addition is by way of another classical formula there is generally a greater degree of response to it than that for an individual modifying material. Where the addition is another formula, and refinement to it has not yet been made, now is perhaps an ideal time to begin the refinement process, again 'making hay when the sun is still shining'.

A difficulty I find, with making additions to a recipe's formulation, is that the period of time additions demonstrate a beneficial response may be shorter than for the second stage refined recipe they are used in conjunction with, requiring me to continue testing the responses to them separately and quite regularly during the time they appear indicated for use, and to not just assume they will be appropriate if the refined recipe benefits the responses. However, if they do prove to consistently work together as a combination, I will combine them for later use.

When identifying any modifying materials, and assessing their optimum therapeutic dose for my own personal use, as with carrying out any part of the refinement process for myself to the recipe's formulation, again I tend to rely on the DICT as my main guide, with the support of several other responses I regularly observe. When working with a patient I am able to observe a variety of other responses in them, to those I am working with for myself, plus I have the added possibility to gain the patient's feedback of response in subjective terms.

When no further response is observable, from testing a particular recipe or any of its components, this is therefore not necessarily the end to the refinement process, as some further modification or addition to this product's design may be possible. A therapeutic recipe modified in some fashion, by way of what else it is prepared in or added to it, always provides an increase in the level of beneficial response as compared to the unmodified version for the same, just as each stage in the refinement process will always benefit the responses beyond the previous stage's recipe formulation.

This process described, in re-assembling the ancient and traditional therapeutic remedies of East Asia to obtain the greater beneficial influence upon the senses and responses, is transferable to working with any therapeutic material or action, at least to some degree. The principles in this are certainly applicable to therapeutically working with materials more indigenous to the region one lives, and maybe even facilitate the successful incorporation of local therapeutic materials into these same traditional recipe formulations, if one were forced or wished to do so, or simply provide the means to utilise locally sourced materials therapeutically. Arguably the processes here described, for working with guidance provided by the senses and responses to make up therapeutic combinations, may somewhat mirror how the peoples of more traditional cultures would have originally gone about selecting and formulating their medicines, although probably using a different set of the responses to observe than used by myself. A colleague, working more with Western herbs as medicine, told me of when she travelled through Peru or Bolivia and meeting up with some local traditional practitioners who were making observation of the pulses to guide them in their selection of remedy. Much of this discussed may also provide a feel to what underlies the roots of Folk Medicines, and possibly even aspects of Shamanistic practices, although I am unable to qualify this opinion from my own experience.

As I develop in this work, on from what I had been doing in my earlier days of practice, I reflect how I then worked differently with the responses yet still my patients and myself gained something from the experience, well at least most of the time, indicating there are potentially many ways to work in this, and that this described is just what I am doing at the moment. Whilst I struggle to develop on from being a relative novice, working with the traditional therapies and medicine of East Asia, without suitably experienced teachers being constantly present to hold my hand as I go, observing the senses and responses has provided me with some form of a guide and connection to what I believe a more experienced practitioner is in practice essentially working with, when all else is taken away, making up for my insufficiencies in practical knowledge and experience. Working with the senses and responses has to be likened to old expression of 'flying by the seat of one's pants'.

I must also point out I am just assuming that seeking the greater response from a therapeutic agent is better than going with something less beneficially inducing of response. I have no evidence in support of this approach, but it is my impression that gaining the greater degree of response can produce the more dramatic and quicker overall improvements in an individual's therapeutic progression. It could however be the case, in terms of the overall influence upon the individual, that there is nothing much more gained by going for the greater response therapeutically, as gauged by the DICT or other responses, and the overall effect still ends up as just the same as when taking or practicing something to provide a lesser degree of beneficial response. Just as taking more of something has the greater response until the optimum therapeutic dose is taken, less may still have affect on the responses sufficient to induce an overall change and improvement in the individual's responses in the longer term. In the end working with achieving less or more response could work out to a similar therapeutic outcome for that person. I think this probably needs my proper consideration, in that I expect to know less than half of picture in this regard, but this could help explain why so many different therapeutic means appear to induce beneficial change.

My observation, through recreating these traditional therapeutic recipes according to the responses, is that there should be nothing within the design's components compromising to the responses, or at least is perceivable as such when applying these, as I have been approaching this work according to an idea that each and every component in these therapeutic recipes should individually demonstrate a benefit for the senses and responses. If one were to be designing anything else, without it needing to be therapeutically beneficial to the responses but just neutral, and be forced into using a component that were to independently compromise the responses, this would perhaps not be a problem if it is not perceivable by the responses within the whole design. However, from my own experiences of testing things containing just traces of a compromising component within their make up, as I have gone on to further refine my senses and responses, I have become more able to perceive things that I was previously unable to clearly make observation of in this regard, and spot an issue. However there is definitely a cut off point for me, within my perceptions, where I can no longer observe any trace of compromise, thinking along the lines of the spread of my perceptive field interacting with the degree of compromise being generated by something, but this is just my impression of what I think may be going on.

Designers, working according to the needs of the senses and responses, need to be especially mindful of coming to, or working from, theoretically based conclusion to predict how the senses and responses will or will not be affected by a particular design, as this can easily lead to oversights generating compromise that the senses and responses may have been able to pick up upon much earlier in the design process. Many seemingly innocuous, but functionally necessary, component additions to a design can very easily be overlooked for their potential of compromise because of the limited degree of their inclusion, or offer of necessary functional benefit. Therefore, unless practicing extreme diligence in applying the senses and responses within the entire design process, it is very easy for compromising components to creep into our designs and lives.

I offer three rather simplistic examples of observations I have made of materials and design compromised by way of the addition of something seemingly insignificant to the product. The first I have mentioned before, being the information labels in clothing. The material of the clothing article, in all its components, could be 100 percent sense and response friendly yet the label, sitting next the skin, induces some level of overall compromise to the article as a result of the label being made from a material compromising to the senses and responses.

The next example is for a sweatshirt I used to wear all the time, with a fancy design printed on it reminding me of a good place I once visited. The fabric was cotton, as far as I was aware a material fine for my own responses and I had chopped out the care label, but I later realised the big design on it was printed in something that, when it was just touched, compromised my responses. It took me a while to figure that one out, as I had been wearing the article for quite a few years until fairly recently. In fact it was actually worn out when I discovered the issue, as I hadn't ever imagined the print could have affected the responses, so assumed it to have been acceptable, but with some back of my mind inkling something was not quite right whenever I wore it. This back of the mind inkling of a thought is very easily over ridden to ignore it, and I'm still trying to learn to act more upon these inklings and test the things around me I may be unsure of when experiencing this sort of a feeling.

My final example is for the fabric linen, about which I had been extremely excited as it is a practical natural material, produced from the fibre of the Flax seed plant and a potential alternative for me to cotton in my life. This was something I was particularly interested in as it seemed to help me 'earth' better through, than cotton, as observable with the responses. In my excitement for the material's potential I ordered all sorts of samples of linen during my 'earthing' phase days, direct from manufacturers and wholesalers, only to then discover some of these samples appeared to compromise my responses by some degree. I even had my wife play a game with me by way of my blind testing them all and indicating which of the samples compromised my responses. Whilst these observations were made quite early on, when my senses were not so refined, it raises the portent matter of ' What else has been done to a material or product during manufacture that may have a compromising influence upon the senses and responses of the user?'

I imagine many people might have some sort of personal wish list for the world of design and manufacture if the opportunity availed them. For me this would be for a more sense and response friendly design to the world I choose to live in, as I cannot seem to function as effectively in the regular world of society without certain things, due to having no access to their sense and response friendly alternatives. If I need to live with these things, consistently compromising of my senses and responses, I have to make myself aware of the consequences of this, applying much of my time to follow practices countering to the compromise. Essentially I cannot function as effectively as I believe I may, with or without these certain things, so find myself in a quandary. Am I going to be better or worse off with those things in my life?

Here is my list of those certain things I am most needing access to in order to more effectively function in the regular world of today's society, plus a couple of things I think need to be the case to be able to live with significantly less compromise to my senses and responses. My Santa Claus wish list.

- A sense and response friendly car, or to have another means of personal conveyance that is not involving a horse.

- A sense and response friendly bicycle and cycle paths.

- Under shorts/pants made from response friendly linen, and without elastin or metals to hold them up.

- A sense and response friendly mobile communication devise (telephone) and portable computer.

- Running shoes, as well as a pair of hiking boots, with soles made of material facilitating me to earth through them, as well as being made completely from response friendly materials.

- Public transport designed to be more sense and response friendly.

- Road surfaces that are not compromising my senses and responses.

- More trees, green spaces, and for nature to be just left to get on with it to a much greater extent.

- Brasiers that do not compromise the responses (for my wife), and response friendly lady under garments.

- To upgrade, or remove from service, all public buildings and areas compromising to the senses and responses of their users.

Most other things I currently see as potentially compromising of my senses and responses can be gotten about if needed whilst still living within regular society. These listed here are what I see as being the most urgently needed in order to live more fully in a sense and response friendly manner. As many, or in fact most, of these on my wish list are quite possibly beyond the realms of foreseeability within my lifetime, and I wish to live now in my own sense and response friendly manner, as and when I choose, I am going to have to limit the incorporation of what I find as compromising somehow or other, whilst continuing to make my contribution within society in an effective manner. I hope we can soon locate what I think is needed for my wife.

New materials are being created all the time. One I was particularly struck by was a fabric, used to make a pair of surf shorts, apparently made from recycled plastic bottles. Someone else was wearing them at the time, so I was only able to literally have a quick feel, but they seemed to test out as fine for my responses. I don't know how sustainable this type of material is, or if it really was as friendly to my senses and responses as it appeared then, but this highlights the added potential for benefit coming from a direction more sustainable as well as friendlier to the senses and responses of the user.

A number of matters have been raised here, as a result of working with the senses and responses, with possible significance to a variety of professional disciplines and interest groups. From the viewpoint of a study of mankind, anthropology concerning our medical roots as one example, once the senses and responses have been reapplied, in navigating one around the natural remedy materials of our ancestors and ancient peoples, the implication behind significant old theories and ideas become clearer and better understood, or equally disproven, through insights provided from observing the responses.

If it has been possible to transmit an idea that observing how we each respond, or react in unconcious ways, to materials is where mankind's future is at, then that must surely be a good thing? However the reality of making changes to suit our sensory findings can be a matter of contention, as it is soon observed how far off track mankind is in this. But, to maintain an enthusiasm for investigating the responses, I reflect how these are a major, yet currently little used, source for insight about how materials affect humans. Where science works backward from making these sorts of observations of the sensory experience, it proves possible to confirm why certain things are found as they are, or identifies the need for new ways of doing things to improve mankind's lot. Ultimately, this leads me to conclude how the basis for doing life needs re-assessing, from the trousers up.

In reflection, when I think about the senses and the responses, I see this is my referring to the senses as the subjective response and the responses as the objective and measurable response, at least on some level. On another level, as may have been inferred within the text of Trousers, the subjective 'senses' are with what we perceive our world, and the more objective 'responses' are the gauge by which to appreciate the depth we are perceiving our immediate world around us. In such way perception becomes measurable as a result of these senses and responses, of which I speak, operating in tandem with each other.

Waiting Through

Man of two souls, how can the two become?
Bathing in fragrance of summer pine,
sucking waters to within,
I die and am reborn.

On route I shed a tear, for myself before I'm gone,
moving toward the shadows that were not there,
shake my head at my old self.

I desired to dance with butterflies, teasing on the wind,
harangued soul passes on, in a breeze across the leaves.
Patience holds more for me than virtue.

Reference bibliography ordered by way of inclusion

Chuang-Tzu: The Inner Chapters, Translated by A.C. Graham, first published 1981 by Allen and Unwin. Reprinted 2001 by Hackett Publishing Company, Inc.

North American Journal of Oriental Medicine, www.NAJOM.org
July 2009 isue, 'Paying attention to the breath', by Kamiya Kazunobu of Toronto, Canada.

Charles Darwin's Letters, Volume I.

Chasing the Dragon's Tail by Yoshio Manaka, with Kazuko Itaya and Stephen Birch, 1995, Paradigm Publications, Brookline, Massachusets.

The Einstein Reader by Albert Einstein, 1956, Citadel Press.

North American Journal of Oriental Medicine, www.NAJOM.org
March 2012 'My Apprenticeship with Dr. Ineon Moon', by Jake Paul Fratkin OMD.

North American Journal of Oriental Medicine, www.NAJOM.org
July 2011 issue, "Tetsuro Saito: Taking Shiatsu to New places" by Cheryl Coull, Victoria, BC, Canada, and "Learning to 'Speak Qi' - Diagnostics and therapeutics in Shin So Shiatsu", by Peter Skrivanic D. Ac, Toronto, Canada.

'Proceedings of the Eighth International People-Plant Symposium' on 'Exploring Therapeutic Powers of Flowers, Greenery and Nature', in Awaji, Japan, in 2004. Edited by E. Matsuo, P.D. Relf, M. Burchett, published by the International Society for Horticultural Science, Acta Horticulturae 790 of June 2008.

Green Nature Human Nature - The Meaning of Plants in Our Lives, by Charles A Lewis, of Morton Arboretum, 1996, published by the University of Illinois Press.

The Experience of Nature - A Psychological Perspective, first published by Cambridge University Press in 1989. Currently published by the Michigan State University book sellers, Ulrich's Bookstore, Ann Arbor, Michigan.

Environmental Psychology for Design, by Dak Kopec, published 2006 by Fairchild Publications Inc.

Listening to the Land - Conversations about Nature, Culture, and Eros, by Derrick Jensen, published 2004 by Chelsea Green Publishing Company.

Dwellings - A spiritual history of the living world, by Linda Hogan, published 1995 by W.W. Norton and Company.

The Book of Medicines, poems by Linda Hogan, published 1993 by Coffee House Press.

The King James Edition Bible.

A clinical Guide to Theory and Practise', written by Otsuka Keisetsu and translated by Gretchen de Soriano & Nigel Dawes, published 2010 by Churchill Livingstone Elsevier Ltd.

'The Texts of Taoism - Part I', translated by James Legge, Dover Publications, 1962, as an unaltered reprint of the work first published by Oxford University Press in 1891, The Tao Te Ching of Lao Tzu and The Writings of Kwang-tze (Chuang-Tzu).

The Doors of Perception by Aldous Huxley, published 1954.

Cognition and Environment - Functioning in an Uncertain World, by Stephen Kaplan and Rachel Kaplan, 1981, published Ulrich's Bookstore, Ann Arbor, Michigan,1981.

Alchemy, Medicine & Religion in the China of A.D. 320, by Ko Hung, translated by James Ware, first published 1966 by the Massachusetts Institute of Technology, published by Dover Publications.

'Five Elements and Ten Stems - Nan Ching Theory, Diagnostics and Practise', by Kiiko Matsumoto and Stephen Birch, published 1983 by Paradigm Publications.

North American Journal of Oriental Medicine, www.NAJOM.org
November 1995 issue, 'Looking Forward', article by Miki Shima, OMD, L.Ac.

East Asian Medicine in Urban Japan by Margaret M Lock, first published 1980, University of California Press

Upcoming works by Shaun Sutton (publication due 2015-2018ish)
(Whilst the titles may change, and the ISBN's will remain, these provide an idea on the theme continuing to be worked along)

Going sense and response friendly.
The 'how toxic are my trousers?' workbook.
ISBN 978-0-9576346-1-9

The workbook supports a structured approach to going more sense and response friendly, covering the steps necessary to break free of theory and convention concerning material selection. The workbook initiates personal documentation of discoveries concerning what the senses and responses select to be lived with, as well as assessing how going more sense and response friendly affects one's life.

Exploring a world at end of the road.
Identifying with the language of nature.
ISBN 978-0-9576346-2-6

How do we know when we have genuinely accessed 'the language of nature' for oursleves? Shaun provides details of ideas and the exercises he makes to access nature's world at the other end of the mind, adding a platter of his own cheesy poetry recording when he may have arrived at this esteemed place in himself.

Out of the no time generation.
A summation of going sense and response friendly.
ISBN 978-0-9576346-3-3

A summation of the experiences of those who have gone more 'sense and response friendly', based upon record obtained from the 'how toxic are my trousers?' workbook. When the senses and responses are utilised; is there a trend to materials selection, what appear to be the challenges at home or the workplace, is there potential for societal or individual gain, and if so where? We come out of the mindset and a world created by our parents' generation, now where to for us?

www.herbpublishing.com

Use for your Notes!

Shaun M Sutton

Use for your Notes!

Use for your Notes!

Shaun M Sutton

Use for your Notes!

www.ingramcontent.com/pod-product-compliance
Lightning Source LLC
Chambersburg PA
CBHW020533270326
41927CB00006B/557